Apples, Carrots and Kale-Oh My!

A Beginner's Guide to Juicing

By

Callie C. Bradford, MS
Certified Holistic Health Coach

Table of Contents

* * *

Apples, Carrots and Kale-Oh My! A Beginner's Guide to Juicing

By Callie Bradford, MS
Callie Bradford is a certified Holistic Health Coach.

Callie Bradford, Founder of Next Generation Fit Kids and Transform 4 Wellness, LLC, brings an inspiring dish of educational, professional and personal achievements to the holistic nutrition table. A successful veteran of the biopharmaceutical industry and Integrated Nutrition Health Coach, Callie is described by industry peers as a "happy and dynamic woman who commands the stage." As a 42 year-old vegan, who has personally conquered both food addiction and chronic disease, Callie is a popular speaker who travels the country to educate women and families on how a healthy lifestyle can combat physical and emotional illnesses naturally. Callie healed herself naturally through whole foods, juicing and cleansing. She was inspired to write this book to help answer some of the common questions people have about how to get started on a new healthy juicing journey. This book lays everything out that you need to know very simply. Callie certainly hopes that this book will help take away some of the mystery of juicing and that it is the catalyst to you living a happy, healthy life!

Introduction

* * *

Do you often wake up in the morning with a sluggish feeling—as if the whole world is weighing down on your shoulders? Does this sluggish, lethargic feeling persist throughout the day, leaving you without energy and drive to complete all your tasks?

Do you have so many things to do but lack the energy and the drive to do all those things? You may have tons of paperwork piled up on your desk, a day's work of recordkeeping to do, or maybe a whole house that must be vacuumed, a mountain of laundry that need your attention, or a playdate with your kids that keeps getting pushed back into your calendar.

Does it already feel like a chore whenever you have to do any of those mentioned above?

Well, if you answered "yes" to any of these questions, then you are one of many Americans who are feeling the same way. When you think about it, it's actually very simple—such problems as those mentioned above can actually be attributed to one single thing: the lack of energy.

Now close your eyes and imagine waking up every day—your mind fresh, your senses alert and your body feeling very light. You have such a great feeling that you know you can take on whatever the days bring you!

Now didn't that feel great?

If just thinking about the potential of what you can achieve with proper diet and nutrition already makes you THAT excited, can you imagine what it would be like to have that kind of feeling all the time? To actually live that life?

Well if you picked up this e-book thinking about how juicing can help you be healthier, more energetic and enthusiastic about life in general, then congratulations! You just made a very important decision—one that can potentially change your life forever.

Welcome to the good life, welcome to the world of juicing!

Chapter 1. Juicing: The Healthier Alternative

* * *

Now that you have made the life-changing decision to go "juicing," there are a few basic things you need to know. Though the term "juicing" already implies what it is all about, there's actually more to it than the ordinary reader would care to know about.

You may have heard about juicing through the local news, through your favorite celebrity who has suddenly become an avid juicing aficionado, through magazines, or through your friends, neighbors or co-workers all swearing by this latest craze. Regardless of the source of information from which you learned about juicing, it is highly likely that you picked up this e-book because you wanted to get substantial and detailed information about juicing before you try it.

THAT is exactly what this e-book is all about!

Certainly, there is a science to it and we would like to help you understand what juicing is all about, how easy it is to incorporate it in your daily habits, and what you stand to gain by making the conscious decision to mind your health and get more out of life through juicing

What is Juicing?

Now, to get on with the discussion, what exactly is "juicing?" How is it different from "smoothing" or even just drinking a glass of natural fruit juice daily?

Simply put, "juicing" originally refers to the act of extracting the juice of out whole fresh fruits and raw, uncooked vegetables and then combining the juices into a drink, which is then taken cold anytime during the day. In the past, we were only used to drinking fresh juice—traditionally either orange or apple—straight out of the carton or a bottle.

Whenever we choose to juice fruits and vegetables, we are actually extracting all the good stuff, leaving only the fibrous pulp and indigestible fiber, which can then be thrown away. What is now left is the pure, natural juice filled with nutrients. When we drink the juice, such nutrients, now available in larger quantities than if we ate the fruits or vegetables whole, can now be easily absorbed by the body.

Popular fruits for juicing include the iniquitous apples as well as berries, citrus, pineapples, cranberries, papaya, and melons, among others. Today, drinking juice is no longer restricted to fruits but now also includes a wide range of vegetables including kale, collard greens, wheatgrass, cucumber, cabbage, swiss chard, leaf lettuce, beets, celery, sweet potato, carrots, broccoli, fennel, kohlrabi greens, and even radishes, to name a few.

In juicing, extracting the juice is typically achieved with the help of high-powered extractors or juicers. Since juicing essentially involves transforming whole fruits and vegetables into liquid, you need an efficient juice extractor or juicer to do the job. Juicing machines for home use typically cost in the range of $40 dollars to over $300 dollars.

What the juicer does is to chop or slice the fruits and vegetables into tiny manageable pieces and then spin these around and around in such a way that the pulp or fiber gets separated from the juice. The pulpy remains are led to a special compartment, while the juice flows out, ready to fill your glass.

If you have no idea where to buy the best juicer or what factors to consider when buying one, the next chapter will help you out. For now, let us focus on juicing and its many benefits.

The Rising Popularity of Juicing

In the past, a small number of devotees have already cultivated a lifestyle that revolves around juicing. However, its popularity surged in the past two years mainly due to the endorsement of popular celebrities, such as Gwyneth Paltrow, Chelsea Handler, Nicole Richie, Alicia Silverstone, Reese Witherspoon, Kim Cattrall, and Blake Lively, to name just a few. These gorgeous, sexy women of all ages have all been spotted toting their favorite "blends" while out in public.

Now if you thought juicing is just for women celebrities, you may be surprised to know that even heartthrobs such as Colin Farrell, Owen Wilson, and Edward Norton have also embraced juicing. Considering that both male and female celebrities have come to enjoy the benefits of juicing, then there is pretty good reason why it has become popular among these health conscious individuals. One way of telling when something has become so popular, and probably addicting, is when even large chain outlets such as Starbucks also begin selling their own healthy blends.

Juicing is also currently making its presence known in the healthy foods market. In fact, the global juices industry has posted annual increase in sales, and with the industry's growth, the annual sales figure is expected to increase by up to US$10.7 billion by 2015.

Although the demand for bottled juice blends compete with other beverages, such as bottled water as well as sports and energy drinks, the thirst for juicing has continued to increase in the last few years. This is mainly due to the increasing demand for healthier alternatives, resulting from heightened awareness for healthy living.

Another indicator that juicing has become very popular these days is that, according to statistics, there has been a 60% increase in the number of juicers being sold in the market for last year alone. What this means is that more and more people are realizing the potential of juicing, not just as a trend, but as an honest-to-goodness way to keep them healthy and fit.

Smoothing, Juicing, What's in a Name?

By now, you may already be familiar about what juicing is and what the juice is supposed to look like when properly executed. However, one question may still be bothering you at this point.

So now we come to the million-dollar question: Is Smoothing the Same as Juicing?

The answer would be "No."

To compare the two, juicing is different from smoothing in that the former uses only the juice while the latter uses all parts of the fruits and vegetables being processed.

In juicing, only the extracted juices of the chosen fruits and vegetables are used and turned into a refreshing drink. This can be achieved in two ways. When using a masticating juicer, the machine masticates or grinds the fruits and vegetables down. As it does so, the juice is slowly extracted and the remaining material is discarded. The final product is a thin, watery liquid that packs all the nutrients from the masticated fruits and vegetables into a few ounces of liquid.

Another kind of juicer, the centrifugal juicer, spins the ground bits of fruits and vegetables. The centrifugal force then separates the liquid from the pulp. The juicer basically produces the same final product—the liquid components of the processes fruits and vegetables.

One advantage of juicing compared with smoothing is that here, you get more of the essential nutrients packed into the liquid. If you are the type of person with a sensitive digestive system that cannot easily digest whole fruits and vegetables, then juicing is definitely the option for you.

Furthermore, removing the fiber from the fruits and vegetables, and ingesting only the good, liquid stuff means that the nutrients are quickly absorbed by your body. This is because fiber is the natural substance that helps the body slowly absorb nutrients from the food we eat.

In addition, you can consume "more" fruits and vegetables when you only drink the juice. However, others would say that the liquid is less filling than a blended smoothie.

In comparison, with smoothing, you dump your fruit and vegetable of choice onto a blender, and then whip everything up until you get a smoothie. Here, both the juice and the pulpy or fibrous parts of the fruits or vegetables are also included in the drink and then ingested.

Using a blender, you can create a final product that is creamier and thicker, simply because the fibers have been incorporated into the drink. However, a smoothie is more filling than juice. Thus, you may have to consume more fruits and vegetables before you can have the same amount of nutrients that you can find in the extracted juice alone.

What Can Juicing Do For You?

Certainly, one of the main reasons why juicing has become so popular these days is that it has so many health benefits and is so convenient to prepare. In a classic case of "Why didn't I think of that before?" many people are slowly becoming juicing devotees simply because the idea is so simple yet so ingenious.

Who would have thought that there was actually a shortcut in enjoying all the health benefits of "eating" fruits and vegetables without exerting effort in cooking and preparing them?

In this part, we will discuss with you some of the most important advantages of juicing as a healthy alternative.

Perhaps to underscore what juicing can do to your body, you may liken the word "juicing" with "supercharging," because this is exactly what you are doing—you are supercharging your body by increasing nutrient intake through drinking pure vitamins, micronutrients, and even enzymes found in fruits and vegetables.

As you do so, you not only avoid the chemicals found in processed food, but also radically initiating wonderful changes in your body, such as boosting your metabolism and reducing or neutralizing your body's acidity levels.

- **Speaking of acidity, stress and even toxins found in our environment can make our bodies more acidic than it should be.** When this happens, our body becomes more conducive to acquiring diseases because our immune system is considerably weakened. However, with juicing, we can restore the normal acidity of our body, thus preventing diseases.

- **Juicing also promotes cell regeneration.** As previously mentioned, high acid levels in the body make it weaker, unable to perform healthy functions such as cell generation. In fact, cancers thrive in bodies that cannot properly regenerate cells. To avoid this, it is best to drink extracted liquid from fruits and vegetables such as beet, lemon, avocado, tomatoes, broccoli, carrots and berries, to name a few.

- **In relation to the above, juicing also prevents premature aging.** High acidity levels in the body increase oxidative stress that lead to age spots and wrinkles. With juicing, you can have fresher, more radiant skin.

- **Vegetables such as cauliflower, broccoli, kale and cabbage contain phtonutrients that include indole-3-carbinol (I3C) and diindolylmethane (DIM).** When you include these in your recipes, you will get the benefits of improved, blood sugar control, and reduced body fat. Hence, one of the most important benefits of juicing is that it helps with weight management.

- **Another major benefit of juicing is that it can help us maintain normal levels of blood pressure.** This is because our arteries become dilated when our body's acidity level is high. If this is the case, then it becomes difficult to control related symptoms of hypertension, arrhythmia, increased blood pressure, and even heart attack resulting from these.

- **Electrolytes, including sodium, calcium, potassium, and magnesium—the stuff found in most fruits and vegetables—help our body function well.** Without these, we may feel less energized and not get the full benefits of a well-functioning body. With juicing, you can increase your intake of fruits and vegetables that contain these electrolytes.

- **You may not know it, but fatty acids actually serve important roles in nerve and brain functioning.** When then metabolism of fatty acid is disturbed, you may be prone to potentially debilitating neurological diseases such as multiple sclerosis. With juicing, you can promote lipid and fatty acid metabolism in your body.

- **Once again, high acidity levels in our body may lead to a poorly functioning circulatory system, wherein there is "corrosion" in the veins, heart tissues and arteries.** This is because the acid in our body weakens the cell wall membranes that make up these tissues. With juicing, you can reduce or neutralize acidity levels in the body to help strengthen the circulatory system.

- **Finally, the normal cells become "sick" and unable to function properly when the body that houses them is acidic.** Drinking the juice of fruits and vegetables that neutralize acidity can help you ensure that more oxygen is delivered to all cells in your body, thus promoting healthier cells.

Doing It The Right Way

With all the benefits listed above, you are probably super excited to try out this healthy alternative. After all, who wouldn't want to feel younger, fresher, have more energy and reduce risk for diseases with something so simple and inexpensive?

Here are some tips to ensure that you are "juicing" in a safe way.

- **Keep in mind that juicing is not a diet in and of itself—you still need to consume over 2000 calories per day so that you still have a balanced diet.**

Although juicing can supercharge your body with much needed phytonutrients, your body still requires sufficient amounts of protein, fat, vitamins, carbohydrates and minerals that you will not necessarily get from just drinking the juice of fruits and vegetables.

- **It is best to drink freshly prepared juice every time.** This is because the juice that you prepare beforehand could develop bacteria once it's been exposed to various pathogens in the environment. Extracted juice that has been left to stand for too long may also have reduced nutritional value, not to mention the fact that it may have an unpleasant taste by then.

- **As mentioned earlier, in juicing, you only drink the liquid component of the fruits and vegetables, the fibrous, pulpy bits are always discarded.** Thus, you may also want to incorporate a small amount of fiber into your diet just to make sure that your digestive system is running well.

- **Finally, though it is pretty obvious, do wash the fruits and vegetables thoroughly before extracting their juice.** Washing them helps remove pesticides or dirt that may be present. At the same time, wash all utensils to be used (including knives, glasses and chopping board). Then, you should also clean the juicer after every use. The manufacturer usually provides cleaning instructions in the manual.

This opening chapter gave you an overview of juicing, its definition and why it is different from smoothing. We also explained the reasons behind its resurging popularity and most of all, we listed down the many benefits you can gain from juicing. The chapter ends with a few smart tips to ensure that you are juicing safely.

The next chapter will be devoted to juicers—how to choose the right one, the factors to consider when choosing one, pricing guide, and so on.

Chapter 2. So Many Juicers So Little Time

* * *

In the previous chapter, we discussed basic information about juicing, specifically, its meaning, how it's different from smoothing, and why it has become popular in recent years. In addition, we also discussed the main benefits of juicing. In this chapter, we shall discuss the next important component of embracing the juicing lifestyle—the juicer.

This chapter is all about juicers. In particular, we shall show you the many different kinds of juicers in the market, factors you need to consider when choosing a juicer, some tips on how to maintain your juicer, and reviews of the top juicers being sold in the market right now. In other words, this chapter shall provide you with important juicer-related information, which brings you closer to a healthier, more energetic lifestyle.

So, What Type of Juicer Should You Buy?

This seems to be the first question that pops up in anyone's mind when coming across the concept of juicing. It is possible that you are reading this e-book right now because you want to find out what kind of juicer you should buy. You may already have an idea about what kind of juicer you want. If you've seen those endless Jack LaLanne infomercials on TV, then there you go, that's a basic juicer.

However, there is no one perfect juicer out there. Just as there are many kinds of fruits and vegetables to mix together to create your own "blends," then there are also many types of juicers available in the market—they differ in size, function, price, and so on. So, for a newbie, how do these juicers differ from one another? How do they compare? How do you know which one suits your lifestyle?

Let us answer these questions one by one, and we shall begin by identifying the basic types of juicers.

Masticating Juicers

Also known as "cold press juicers," masticating juicers derive their name from the word "masticate," which means to soften, crush, or grind food. Basically, masticating juicers produce juice by crushing and pressing fruit and vegetables. As in humans, a basic masticating juicer "chews" fruits and vegetable fibers, breaks them up and produces juice with greater yield. The juicer does this with sharp blades that first cut up the fruits and vegetables, before they are pressed down to extract juice from them.

The masticating juicer is the best choice for someone who really likes fresh juice, is into cleansing, and would also like to make other slow-pressed food products with the masticating juicer. This type of juicer is also perfect for those who wish to extract the most minerals and nutrients from the fruits and vegetables that they process.

Advantages/Disadvantages of a Masticating Juicer

One of the most important advantages of a masticating juicer is that this type of juicer is more efficient than other types because they produce more juice from the same amount of fruits and vegetables than other juicers. Thus, for example, you get more apple juice from two apples from a masticating juicer than from a centrifugal juicer processing the same number of apples.

In addition, masticating juicers can extract juice from virtually all kinds of fruits and vegetables. In fact, some types of masticating juicers, such as the single gear juicers can even extract juice from traditionally difficult vegetables to extract, such as spinach, parsley, lettuce, wheatgrass, herbs, and other kinds of green and leafy vegetables.

Second, while extracting juice, masticating juicers do not produce greater amounts of heat and froth as much as the other types. Because it must operate at a slow speed compared with a centrifugal juicer (which has to run in high speed), a masticating juicer is capable of keeping nutrients from the fresh ingredients because of the moderate temperature they have during extraction. It is also for this reason why juice extracted through a masticating juicer has a longer shelf life, thus reducing wastage.

Third, masticating juicers can be used for other purposes such as making thick sauces, ice cream, sorbet, baby foods, and even nut milk or nut butter. Some of the more expensive ones can even help you make small bread sticks and pasta.

In terms of disadvantage, masticating juicers work slowly and surely, hence, it may not be ideal for those who are on the go and want to extract juice quickly. Furthermore, masticating juicers also tend to be more on the expensive side compared with other juicers. However, we are sure that the advantages we have listed above far outweigh the disadvantage brought about by a more expensive price tag.

Centrifugal Juicers

Now let's go to the second type of juicer, which is the centrifugal juicer. If the masticating or slow press juicer is more on the expensive side, then the centrifugal juicer is more popular because it is more reasonably priced. The reason behind this is that it possesses one of the simplest mechanisms compared with other more complex juicers.

Centrifugal juicers employ a rapidly spinning blade that spins against a filter, which is responsible for separating fruit and vegetable juice from their original, pulpy, and fibrous state. From its name, we can tell that the centrifugal juicer utilizes centrifugal force to extract juice from your chosen fruits and vegetables. Centrifugal force refers to the force generated when something moves away from a center or an axis. In this case, the fruits and vegetables are sliced, ground to a pulp and then spun around so that the juice is separated from the juicy pulp. The juice drips down one chute, while the remaining pulpy fibers go down another chute.

Generally, centrifugal juicers come in designs that feature large chutes that can accommodate smallish fruits, such as apples and oranges. Thus, this is perfect for people on the go—people just like you—since you can save a few precious minutes of your time cutting and dicing the fruits and vegetables before you can juice them..

The centrifugal juicer is an excellent choice for those who don't have a lot of money to spend on the more efficient, but expensive masticating juicers. This is also ideal for people who don't mind getting fewer amounts of nutrients per processing as long as they are able to extract enough juice for drinking.

Did you know that a centrifugal juicer also works best for processing fruits ad vegetables for cooking and baking purposes? If, aside from juicing, you are also passionate about cooking and juicing, then the centrifugal juicer is the best choice

Advantages/Disadvantages of a Centrifugal Juicer

As mentioned above, one of the advantages of using centrifugal juicers is that it can rapidly and quickly extract juice. Hence, this is the perfect choice for people just like you who may want to have their juice on the go. The centrifugal juicer is also perfect for extracting juice from tougher and harder parts of fruits and vegetables, such as pineapple cores, since a centrifugal juicer features steel blades that cut and slice fruits ad vegetables before the juice is extracted.

Another advantage is that centrifugal juicers are less expensive than their more complex, high-end counterparts such as the masticating or slow-press juicers. Thus, if you are a newbie juicer and want to experiments for the first few months, then buying a starter centrifugal juicer is the perfect, commitment-free way to get started.

Yet another advantage is the fact that you can use your centrifugal juicer to process other ingredients for cooking and baking purposes. Hence, buying a centrifugal juicer is actually like buying two or three machines for the price of one!

In terms of disadvantages, one concern lies in the fact that the rapidly spinning action that is responsible for separating juice from the pulp is the same action that generates excess heat. Such heat can reduce or kill the enzymes from the juice you are producing. Hence, the nutrient value of the final product is lessened compared with what you get with a masticating juicer.

Meanwhile, centrifugal juicers may also produce less liquid ounce of juice from your chosen fruits and vegetables compared with masticating juicers. This is because the high-speed, rotation is not efficient enough to extract 100% of the liquid from the fruits and vegetables. In fact, the pulpy byproduct of the centrifugal juicer is still moist, proof that not all of the liquid is separated from the pulp.

In addition, while a centrifugal juicer can also be used to extract juice from green leafy vegetables. However, the yield is considerably less than that of the masticating juicer.

Finally, when using a centrifugal juicer, the shelf life of the final product may also be shorter because juice extracted from this type of juicer tends to have more oxygen in it. Since the very basic operation of a centrifugal juicer requires high speed spinning action, this process aerates the liquid, incorporating oxygen into the final product. The generated oxygen bubbles lead to oxidation that, in turn, leads to quick spoilage of the juice.

Twin-Gear Juicers

Finally, the last type of juicer we will feature here is the twin-gear or triturating juicer. According to juicing experts, of all the juicers available in the market, this is the most efficient and has the best features. Of course, these come at a hefty price tag. Nevertheless, devotees believe that the expensive price of a twin gear juicer is outweighed by the many advantages you can get from this product.

How does it work exactly?

A twin gear juicer works in a similar way to the masticating juicer. Basically, it presses sliced fruits and vegetables using two interlocking gears that roll continuously, hence the name "twin gear." The difference with the masticating juicer, however, is that the twin gear juicer works at an even slower speed than the masticating juicer.

With a super slow speed, the twin gear juicer is capable of breaking open even the tougher cell walls, thus releasing more nutrients, enzymes, vitamins, and minerals from whatever it is you are juicing.

A twin gear juicer is also called the "triturating juicer." Literally, "trituration" refers to the process of crushing or grinding food into ultra fine particles. Hence, what the triturating juicer or twin gear juicer does is to crush and grind fruits and vegetables intro extremely fine particles so that everything is turned into juice.

Juicing experts believe the basic features of the twin gear juicer comprise its many advantages. For instance, the twin gear juicer can extract juice of very high quality, it operates at low speed thus producing less noise, it can be used for purposes other than juicing, and , it can produce greater yield per fruit or vegetable,

With the latter feature mentioned above, you can tell that the twin gear juicer is more efficient because the pulpy byproduct it produces as it separates the liquid from the fibers is the driest of all, in comparison with the byproducts generated by the masticating juicer or by the centrifugal juicer.

If these reasons do not convince you of the superior juicing power of the twin gear juicer, then do read on as we present the other advantages of the twin gear juicer in the next segment of this chapter.

Advantages/Disadvantages of a Twin-Gear Juicer

As mentioned above, the twin gear juicer has so many advantages, let's take a look at some of them.

First, the twin gear juicer is considered the most efficient of all types of juicer because it is capable of producing more liquid ounce of juice from a variety of fruits and vegetables compared with a masticating juicer or a centrifugal juicer. The twin gear juicer is capable of extracting precious liquid even from small or tough leafy vegetables such as the popular wheatgrass, kale, spinach, pine needles, and a whole lot of other herbs and vegetables.

Second, it is relatively easier to use a twin gear juicer because it has a self-feeding action, which sucks in soft fruits and leafy vegetables. This self-feeding action is due to the twin gears that roll inward while crushing the fruits and vegetables fed into it. In case you need to juice relatively tougher produce, such as carrots, radishes, or even apples, you may need to slice them up into smaller, thinner, and more manageable parts.

Third, a twin gear juicer turns at a slower speed than the masticating juicer or centrifugal juicer. Thus, there is less aeration or incorporation of oxygen into the final liquid product. What this means is that you can store your juice longer for up to 36 hours because the juice will not spoil easily. The slow speed of the two gear juicer also means that it generates less heat than other types of juicers. Thus, you get maximum amounts of nutrients, enzymes, and other good stuff from your fruits and vegetables.

Fourth, as mentioned before, a twin gear juicer can be used for other purposes, making it an excellent investment in the kitchen. For example, it can be used to easily grind and crush tough produce such as apples, pumpkins and carrots, as well as easily crush soft ingredients at the same time. Thus, you can use your twin gear juicer not just to extract high quality juice, you can also use it for making baby food, ice cream, butter, sorbet, and even pasta and bread.

Finally, a twin gear juicer is a heavy-duty machine. What you lose in counter-top space, you gain in terms of performance, stability and durability.

In terms of disadvantages, the first obvious disadvantage is that it is quite pricey, with prices ranging anywhere from $500 to $1,000. It is also a bit more complex than a masticating juicer or the relatively simpler centrifugal juicer, hence, it is not ideal for beginner juicers.

Finally, there may be a considerable prep time involved in extracting tough produce since you will need to slice them so that they can easily be fed into the chute. If you are the type who want to have their juice fast, fresh, and easy then the twin gear juicer may not be the best option for you.

Some Factors You Need To Consider When Choosing A Juicer

As with other major purchases, you need to consider several important factors that can help you buy the right product. In this case, before you go out and buy a juicer, it would be a great idea if you knew about their basic features and operations. This is because varied types of juicers can also influence many things, such as what kinds of fruits and vegetables you can juice, how much juice you can produce, how fresh the juice can last, and so on.

In this part of the chapter, we shall break down this important decision into several key factors that you need to look into. As you go through the list, do keep your preferences in mind so that, hopefully, by the end of the segment, you would have already made the right choice. Then you can hop on over to our reviews to see if any of those juicers suit you.

Your Juicing Program

The first factor you need to consider before buying a juicer is your overall juicing program. Here, you need to ask yourself a few questions:

- Are you a beginner or an expert?
- Are you just experimenting or willing to make a commitment to the juicing lifestyle?
- What kinds of juicing blends are you going to try?
- Are you only going to use it for fruits only, for vegetables only, or for both?

Depending on your answers to the questions above, then you will be able to narrow down your choices and ultimately select the best juicer that suits your needs and your lifestyle.

First of all, are you a beginner or an expert juicer? Perhaps more readers belong to the first category, which why you are reading this e-book in the first place. If you are a beginner, then you may want to buy a simple, no-frills machine that can do the job quickly and efficiently.

Second, if you are a beginner, then it is highly likely that you are still in the experimenting stage. What this means is that you have not yet established a preference for fruits only, vegetables only or a juice that combines both. If you are not yet sure of your preferences then it may be better not to invest a huge amount if money on a more expensive juicer only to find that you don't have the time to operate it or the patience to clean its many parts.

However, if you are bent on going all out, and plan to use the juicer to extract juice from virtually all kinds of fruits and vegetables, while gaining maximum yield and efficiency, then we recommend that you choose a twin-gear juicer. This way, your investment will have great returns in the form of more amounts of extracted, high quality juice that can be stored for a longer time.

Ease of Use

In relation to the items mentioned above, ease of use is another important consideration. Here, you may need to ask yourself a few more questions before making that final decision.

- Do you prefer ease of use or efficiency?
- Does your schedule allow you to indulge in slow-press juicers or not?
- Do you prefer a juicer that is easy to clean and operate?
- Do you prefer a simple machine or a complex one?

If you are the type of person who is on the go and wants to have her juice fast, fresh and quick, then may want to consider getting a centrifugal user. This is because the centrifugal juicer allows you to extract juice in mere seconds! Unlike the slower masticating juicer or triturating juicer, which operate on a slower speed, you can immediately get fresh juice with a centrifugal juicer in no time.

In terms of features, a centrifugal juicer also has a simpler design that uses fewer components. In comparison, the two other slow-press types of juicers have more parts and more complex designs that a new user may find bewildering. Furthermore, a more complex design means more parts to clean and maintain. Hence, a very busy person may not appreciate a masticating or twin gear juicer.

Price and Cost Consideration

Last but not least in our list of major factors to consider is, of course, the price factor. It is not easy to spend hard-earned money on something you are not 100% sure of. Thus, before setting out to buy any kind of juicer—especially the more expensive ones, you may need to answer the following questions:

- What is your budget?
- Do you want to maximize the nutrients from fruits and vegetables using a high-end juicer or are you willing to sacrifice this for a less-expensive juicer?

First of all, it's your budget that is going to dictate what kind of juicer to get. Juicers range from a few hundred to a few thousand dollars. Which one should you get depends on your budget.

Usually, the more efficient slow-press juicers, such as the masticating juicer and the twin gear juicer, are more efficient and have many parts that help maximize the amount of juice produced per extraction. These kinds of juicers usually have more complex operations, more parts, sturdier materials and are, therefore, more expensive. On the one hand, if you are ready to commit to a juicing lifestyle and if money is not a consideration, then we would suggest that you go all out and buy the more expensive but efficient juicers out there.

On the other hand, if your budget is limited and you are looking for something that is easier to use, has a simpler mechanism, and not to difficult to maintain, then you can go for the less expensive alternatives that still have the capability to juice with mid-level efficiency, but guarantee fresh juice in mere seconds.

Some Reviews of the Top Juicers in the Market

Now that we have laid down the basics, as well as provided you with a list of three important factors to consider when buying a juicer, let us take a look at some of the recommended juicers per type and price range.

Centrifugal Juicer - Philips 1861

The Philips 1861 is a good choice for those who are looking for a dependable centrifugal juicer. At $170, it does not require too much commitment from the buyer while still delivering efficiently—enough to turn a beginner to a juicer pro in a number of days.

This award-winning product features a brushed aluminum body that is not only to clean but also looks good on any kitchen countertop. When you look inside, you will find that most of its parts are made of plastic, what this means is that clean up is so easy! Just remove the parts, pop them into the dishwasher and you're done!

In terms of features, it has a wide chute that can accommodate whole fruits. Thus, there is virtually no need to slice or cut up fruits before extraction. This product also offers two kinds of speed levels—one for softer and tender fruits, and another for tougher produce that are more difficult to juice.

Advantages	Disadvantages
Speed	Juice cannot be stored for longer period
Reasonable price	Could be noisy
Almost zero prep time	Yields lower liquid ounce of juice
Easy to clean and maintain	No citrus attachment

Masticating Juicer - Matstone 6 in 1

At $300, the Matstone 6 in 1 Juicer is definitely a bit more expensive than the common centrifugal juicer. However, the added cost simply means that you get more features and, therefore, more benefits from this machine.

First, the Matstone 6-in-1 Juicer can extract high-quality juice from a variety of fruits and vegetables. Aside from that, it can even be used for making pasta, baby food, ice cream, sorbet, butter, and so on. If you are also a kitchen queen aside from a juicer pro, then this product is a great option.

Because this juicer is a masticating juicer, it is capable of producing more juice with higher quality because the operation does not generate heat that can kill off enzymes and reduce the nutritional value of your juice. At the same time, juice can be stored for up to two days—definitely longer than the shelf life of juice extracted through a centrifugal juicer.

Finally, the Matstoine 6-in-1 Juicer is also easy to clean and maintain, while still being able to extract juice with far greater efficiency than the centrifugal juicer. Hence, you get the best of both worlds with this product.

Advantages	Disadvantages
Can extract juice from wheatgrass	Pricier than centrifugal juicers
Can be used for other cooking purposes	Smaller feeding chutes
Juice can be stored for up to 2 days	More complex and has many parts
Quiet motor	Slow juicing "action"

Twin Gear Juicer - Green Star 2000

As we have mentioned earlier, twin gear triturating juicers are the most efficient of all juicers out there. They produce more liquid ounce of juice from the same number of fruits and vegetables compared with their counterparts.

A representative product, the Green Star 2000, is a prime example of an excellent twin gear juicer. At $550, this is certainly the pricier one of the bunch. However, it is also packed with so many features that will surely convince you that you made the right investment.

One benefit of using this juicer is that it is capable of producing rich, pure, and clean fruit and vegetable juice. Its magnetic and bioceramic technology delays oxidation, which in turn, allows the juicer to extract juice that can be stored for up to two days. Thus, if you are a serious juicer who must have her juice all day everyday, then this is a practical choice for you.

Another thing that makes the Green Star 2000 perfect for pro juicers is that it can extract juice from vegetables that are traditionally difficult to juice, especially those with tough fibers. Thus, this juicer broadens the range of fruits and vegetables that can be included in your recipes.

Advantages	Disadvantages
Can be used for other cooking purposes	Pricier than other types of juicers
Produces rich, high-quality juice	Slow juicing "action"
Juice can be stored for up to 2 days	Cannot be used to juice pineapple
Quiet motor	
Easy to clean and maintain	
Can be used to juice wheatgrass and other	

leafy vegetables	

With this chapter, we hope to have provided you with comprehensive and detailed information about juicers. Primarily, we included information about the main types of juicers, factors to consider before buying a juicer, and some information about the most talked about juicers per type and price range.

We hope that the information found here can help you decide on what juicer to get so that you can begin your transition to a healthier lifestyle via juicing!

Chapter 3. Preparing to Juice

* * *

I n the previous chapter, we presented an overview of important details you need to know before buying a juicer. The previous chapter discussed the various types of juicers, factors to consider, and some details on the most talked about juicers per type and price range. We also included some recommendations for each type of juicer, listing down their advantages and disadvantages to further help you decide.

In Chapter 3, we will now get deeper into the world of juicing as, this time, we will be discussing several things that pertain to the process of juicing itself, including the selection of the rights combinations of fruits and vegetables, health considerations, ensuring balanced flavor, preparation and storage, as well as other practical tips

Choosing the Right Fruits and Vegetables

First of all, juicing is supposed to be seamlessly incorporated into your existing diet habits and preferences. In other words, rather than totally overhaul your diet habits, juicing should enhance and improve what you have been doing so far.

There are two reasons why you need to carefully plan how you should introduce juicing into your diet program. Physiologically speaking, you don't want to shock your body by suddenly introducing rich and potent juice into your system on a regular basis. This shock may have detrimental rather than good effects on your body.

Psychologically speaking, you may already be accustomed to certain flavors, tastes, and textures in your preferred foods. The sudden introduction of juice that you may never have tasted before may condition your mind that it does not taste good, making it difficult for you to enjoy each glass of extracted juice. If it's not enjoyable, then what's the point right?

To help introduce juicing into your lifestyle, it would be better if you start with the proper selection of fruits and vegetables to juice. Depending on your preference, nutritional needs and discipline, you will be able to narrow down you selection to a few choice fruits and vegetables to incorporate into your diet. Here are a few tips to keep in mind.

Tip#1 - Start with something sweet.

It is important that you start off with sweet tasting fruits and vegetables. These include apples and carrots. Specifically, carrots are sweet enough to complement the bitterness of some fruits and vegetables while apples can also serve as the perfect base for when you decide to include more bitter leafy vegetables.

However, you must keep in mind that too much sugar or fructose in your juice can feed harmful yeast and other organisms that, in turn, lead to several problems. These include fatigue, excessive weight gain, upset stomach, and so on.

Tip#2 - Gradually incorporate vegetables.

So as not to shock your system as well as your taste buds, slowly incorporate vegetables once you have grown accustomed to drinking high-powered juice everyday. As you use the more familiar carrots and apples as your juice base, you can then add vegetables gradually until you get used to the taste.

Although there is no doubt that green leafy vegetables, such as kale, lettuce and mustard greens, do wonders for your health. However, some people think their taste is not desirable, especially for newbie juicers. In order to get the healthy benefits of drinking extracted juice from these vegetables, mix them up with more familiar "tastes" that you already prefer. This helps you get accustomed to the flavor slowly until you become more comfortable drinking their juice.

Tip#3 - Keep this ratio in mind: 2-1-1.

Let's admit it, it can be very overwhelming trying to figure out what fruits and vegetables to juice, let alone determine the right amounts for each. To help you with this, perhaps this is a good number to start: 2-1-1. Consider it your code to unlocking the enjoyable and certainly healthy world of juicing!

Well, of course what we mean is as follows: 2 root vegetables, 1 leafy vegetable, 1 watery vegetable.

For the root vegetables, try the small variants like carrots and beets to ensure a power punch of antioxidants to your drink. Carrots, of course, add sweetness to the final blend. If you want to add fruit, you can substitute it with apples or kiwis.

For the leafy vegetable, try to add 1 variant, such as broccoli, kale, collard greens, and so on. Then to add to the whole mix, you can add 1 water-rich vegetable, such as cucumber or celery, to add vitamins into the mix and to ensure a smooth final product. You can then add mint or other herbs to make the drink more refreshing

Ensuring Balanced Flavor

As we have mentioned earlier, it is important to prepare and accustom yourself to the tastes and flavors of various combinations of fruits and vegetables. Juicing is not just about simply extracting juice from produce. This is also about being able to maximize the health benefits from juicing without sacrificing taste and flavor.

At the same time, finding the right balance of fruits and vegetables—in terms of variants and quantities—is not just a fun process, it will also ultimately determine whether juicing can become an integral part of your dietary habits.

Tip#1 - Choose the right sweeteners.

If you need to sweeten your juice but do not like to use carrots, then you can add apples instead. Specifically, Granny Smith apples are best for this purpose because they are not so sweet, a little bit sour, and better able to complement the flavors of extracted vegetable juice.

To balance the flavor, you can also add some lime or lemon juice so that the juice can also have a refreshing and cleansing function. The acidity of citrus juices can also induce healthy BM in the morning.

Tip#2 - Find the right formula.

As we have mentioned before, juicing is supposed to be a fun activity, not to mention a beneficial feature of anyone's diet program when properly followed. Some experts that a good juice contains some or all of the following flavors: sweetness, a tart taste, an earthy taste, a refreshing twist, and some hint of herbs and spices.

Part of the fun of juicing is finding the right mix of flavors that you can incorporate into your juicing program. Here's a quick reference that you can use whenever you are looking for the right fruits and vegetables to provide you with the flavor you are looking for. Feel free to clip it and place it on your fridge.

Flavor/Taste	Examples
Earthy (roots)	Carrots, beets, parsnips, and turnips
Earthy (green leafy vegetables)	Dandelion, lettuce, broccoli, kale, spinach, arugula, chard, mustard greens, sorrel
Sweet	Pears, apples, melons, oranges, kiwis, berries, grapes, mangoes, grapes, pineapples
Refreshing	Limes and lemons
Watery	Celery, cucumbers, tomato, melons, fennel
Herbs	Parsley, mint, cilantro, basil,
Spicy	Ginger, mild peppers

Tip#3 - Don't be afraid to experiment.

As we have mentioned earlier, juicing should be fun! Thus, feel free to experiment on what tastes and flavors suit your taste. There is no bible as to what is the right combination to achieve the best nutrient content and flavor. At best, all we can offer are just suggestions. In the end, it's still up to you because it will be your body that's going to determine whether something is right or is not right for you.

Just remember, don't start right away with the heavy duty, hardcore juicing staples, such as kale, if you have not yet grown accustomed to its taste. There is nothing wrong with starting with familiar fruits and vegetables, such as apples, tomatoes, kiwis, and so on.

If the juice is a bit bitter, you can more apple slices; if the juice is too sweet, then add lime to give it an extra zing! Don't be afraid to experiment, this is the only way that you can find the perfect combination that suits you!

Juicing Your Way to a Healthy Body

You may very well be holding this book right now because you believe juicing is the best way by which to improve your health. You may also be interested in losing weight, and in this regard, juicing is also one of the best ways to achieve that goal.

In this part of the book, let us discuss related information as to how juicing can promote good health, increase your energy, maximize your nutrient intake, and help you manage your weight.

All About Fruits and Vegetables

One of the common mistakes made by newbie juicers is that they believe simply dumping fruits and vegetables into the juicer, extracting their juice, and drinking the liquid is already a health-promoting habit in and of itself. Unfortunately, you also need to avoid some fruits, or at least reduce the amounts, so that you can also avoid several problems related to their excessive intake.

For example, some studies found that increased fruit juice intake may be related to an increase in risk for type 2 diabetes. In addition, sugar found in fruits, called fructose, can form as triglycerides that affect the liver and increase insulin resistance.

Meanwhile, those with low blood sugar level condition or hypoglycemia can also benefit from juicing, especially when you go green, that is, when you prioritize drinking green vegetable juices.

Again, simply drinking extracted fruit juice may be harmful if you drink too much. To avoid this, minimize these sweet fruits and increase your intake of vegetables that can balance such negative effects.

Weight Management

One of the reasons why juicing has become popular these days is that many people, including celebrities, swear by its ability to help them lose weight. If you are into weight loss or simple weight management, you can certainly benefit from juicing.

First of all, the whole idea of juicing is supercharging your system with the much needed nutrients packed into a single glass of liquid goodness. With the concentrated nutrients already present in the juice, there is no longer a need to consume more foods, simply because the nutrients are already in the juice—ready to drink anytime.

Second, depending on the combination of fruits and vegetables, juice blends or juice cleanses can make you feel full. With the feeling of having a full stomach, you no longer have the familiar craving for other foods, the excessive consumption of which can help you gain weight, and fast!

However, you also need to keep in mind that not all sweet fruits are ideal for juicing. Some of them may lead to diabetes and other conditions. To start your diet program, you may want to drink at least 8 ounces of juice a day. As you progress, you may increase your intake and experiment further.

Fiber Is Still Good For You!

Another common mistake first time juicers make is that they think the fibrous byproduct of their juicers have no nutritive value. Hence, they often throw this away and not give it a second thought.

If you are thinking of the same thing, then you need to stop right there!

Studies have shown that even though an individual consumes extracted juice on a regular basis, he or she still needs to eat whole fruits and vegetables to maintain an ideal diet. A diet consisting of 100% juice, no matter how supercharged each glass is, is not a good diet.

In this way, even experts agree that people who juice still need to have fiber into their diet. One good way to reintroduce some fiber back into your diet, you can add a little bit of the fiber produced by your juicer into the juice you are drinking.

Preparation

In terms of the right way to prepare your juice, again, there is no standard universal way of preparing extracted juice. Aside from the strict rule of following your juicer instruction manual, all other things that are covered by preparation—peeling, cutting, washing, and so on—are entirely dependent on each person.

To peel or not to peel, that is the question. If you are unsure whether you need to peel something or not, then check your juicer manual. Some juicers cannot process the tough skin of some fruits and vegetables. If your juicer can handle it, and if you prefer keeping the skin (and the nutrients) intact, then make sure that the produce is organic and grown without pesticides.

Certainly, there is a need to thoroughly wash the produce and the utensils you will be using when extracting juice. If you don't wash them thoroughly, the fruits and vegetables may still have pesticides, or worse, foreign bodies that can get into your juice. Washing also helps prevent bacterial contamination in your drink.

Storage and Other Tips

Once you have successfully extracted juice from your fruit and vegetable selection, you may find yourself asking the following questions: When should I drink the juice? Can I store it for a few hours or a few days? How shall I drink it—cold, warm, room temperature? If you too are asking the same questions, then check out the storage tips we have compiled:

- Ensure that your container can be sealed tight and does not have extra air space inside.

- Fresh, extracted juice is best consumed within 20 minutes after extraction. Depending on your juicer, however, you may be able to store juice longer from six hours after juicing (masticating juicers) to up to 48 hours in the fridge (twin gear juicers).

- The juice should be taken when it is at room temperature. Experts say that this is the optimal temperature by which you can drink it. If you have prepared and stored juice beforehand, you can take out the container and let it stand for a few minutes to even out the temperature before drinking it.

- Experts suggest that you swish the juice around in your mouth before gulping it down. As the juice mixes with your saliva, this process stimulates the digestion process, which is crucial to the body's ability to process the nutrients in the juice.

- It may be helpful if you drink your juice with an empty stomach. This way, your body can absorb the nutrients and all the good stuff found in your glass of extracted juice.

- In relation to the above, drink your most potent juices at the start of the day when you need a lot of complex carbohydrates to produce energy that you need for the day's tasks.

- Though some people believe that drinking acidic citrus juice in the morning may upset your stomach, this may not actually be true in most cases.

There you go! Some more important information you need to know, this time, in relation to the process of juicing itself. Let's see, we have already taught you all about juicers—what to choose, how to choose them, and how to check them. Then in this chapter, we taught you the basics of preparing your juice—from choosing the proper ingredients, ensuring flavor, tips on preparing and storing, and so on.

Congratulations, you are well on your way to being an expert juicer. So what's next then? Well, it's now time to buy the ingredients and check out recipes for juicing. The next chapter will help you navigate through this task. Are you ready? Let's move on to the next chapter and let's go shopping!

Chapter 4. Let's Go Shopping!

* * *

In the past three chapters we have discussed several aspects of juicing that any juicing newcomer must know of—from an overview of what juicing is all about, to a discussion of different types of juicers, down to the basic details about preparing your juice, such as proper ingredient selection, ensuring flavor, preparation and storage tips and so on.

In this new chapter, we will be covering more specific aspects related to fruits and vegetables—the two core components of juicing. Here, our goal is to share with you some useful knowledge, and of course, some practical tips specially related to shopping for produce, what you need to know before setting out to buy fruits and vegetables, some detailed health factors that you need to consider, and so on.

The Shopping List

By now, you must be very excited to get started with your juicing program. But before that, let us tackle the next important step before you can fully juice your way to good health. We are talking about shopping, of course! You cannot start your program if you don't have the fruits and vegetables—along with herbs and other produce—that you will need for your juice.

In this part of Chapter 4, we will share some tips on how to choose the right kinds of fruits and vegetables based on several key factors. Though it can be quite bewildering at first, being armed with the right kind of information will help you choose the right kinds of produce depending on your goal, thus helping you maximize your juicing experience.

What Do You Prefer?

First things first, you need to be able to identify your preference, which will guide you in choosing the right kinds of fruits and vegetables to put in your shopping cart. Regardless of whether you are an expert or new to the world of juicing, you will definitely develop your own set of preferences as you go along. If you have no idea where to start, do read on as we explain a few basic details to help you shop for produce.

Just as in eating food, juicing also follows one basic rule: go with what tastes good! Of course, this is a relative subject because what tastes good for some may not taste as good for the others. If you are new to juicing, it would be best to start with common fruits and vegetables, such as apples, carrots, citrus, and so on. Starting a juicing program with familiar-tasting fruits and vegetables can help your body and your taste buds adapt to the new sensation of drinking extracted juice.

Later on, when you body grows accustomed to the taste of nutrient-rich extracted juice, you can incorporate new stuff into your diet, such as green leafy vegetables, or juicing mainstays like cucumber, green snap beans, radishes, and squash, to name a few.

As you go along, keep a list of combinations that taste good and those that you body can accept (meaning you are able to drink their juice without adverse reactions). However, before concocting your recipes, it may be a good idea to consult your doctor first so that you can cross out fruits and vegetables that may contain elements that can be bad for your body. Here's a juicing cheat sheet that you can follow.

If you want to….	Try to combine…
Dispel excess salts, nourish the bladder and kidney	Pineapple, Apple, Watermelon
Regulate sugar content	Pear and Banana
Prevent constipation	Banana, Pineapple, Milk
Improve skin complexion	Apple, Cucumber, Kiwi
Improve skin texture and moisture	Orange, Ginger, Cucumber
Decrease blood pressure, fight oxidization	Carrot, Apple, Pear, Mango
Prevent cancer, reduce cholesterol, and eliminate stomach upset and headache	Apple, Cucumber, Celery
Improve skin complexion and eliminate bad breath	Tomato, Carrot, Apple
Rich in Vit. C and B2; increase cell activity and strengthen immunity	Honeydew, Grape, Watermelon, Milk
Boost and cleanse system	Carrot, Ginger, Apple
Rich in vitamin C, E, Iron; improve skin complexion and metabolism	Papaya, Pineapple, Milk
Avoid bad breath and reduce internal body heat	Bitter gourd, Apple, Milk

Organic Vs. Non-Organic Produce

You may already be familiar with produce labeled as non-organic and organic, with the main difference being the way such produce have been grown. Non-organic produce are grown in the traditional way, meaning tons of pesticide, fungicides fertilizers, herbicides, soil conditioners, and the like have been used to grow them. Meanwhile, organic produce may be more expensive but these have been grown with little to no pesticide, thus ensuring higher and safer quality.

In contrast, organic farming uses sustainable and renewable techniques to encourage crop yield, preserve soil and water, and reduce negative environmental impact. These techniques include crop rotation and using mulch, compost, and other natural fertilizers and weed inhibitors to feed the soil and control bugs and insects.

For the purpose of juicing, it would be better if you buy organize produce simply because you want to prevent toxic those chemicals from getting into your juice. According to the Environmental Working Group, as you navigate your way through the produce section, keep in mind the so-called Dirty Dozen and the Clean Fifteen produce. If, for some reason, you cannot buy organic produce in your area (maybe due to the lack of options, low budget, etc.), then avoid the Dirty Dozen. However, you can still safely consume the Clean Fifteen because they have been proven the have the least amount of pesticides.

Dirty Dozen	Apples, celery, strawberries, peaches, spinach, nectarines, grapes, bell peppers, potatoes, blueberries, lettuce, kale/collards
Clean Fifteen	Onions, corn, pineapples, avocado, asparagus, peas, mangoes, eggplant, cantaloupe, kiwi, cabbage, watermelon, sweet potatoes, grapefruit, mushrooms

Source: http://www.ewg.org

The Top Ten Fruits and Vegetables for Juicing

Now that you are familiar with some of the produce that you will need to start juicing. These fruits and vegetables, when combined, help us get the greatest amount of nutrients and the maximum benefits from our juicing program.

Indeed, according to Ashley Koff, a registered dietitian with celebrity clients, *"What's so wonderful about juicing is that it gives you the opportunity to introduce foods into your diet you wouldn't normally eat."*

With this in mind, let us take a look at the Top 10 popular fruits and vegetables meant for juicing.

- **Carrots.** Rich in beta-carotene; excellent base that can mask the strong taste of green leafy vegetables such as kale
- **Kale.** Rich in iron and folate
- **Wheatgrass.** Rich in Vitamins C, E, and K; has high cellulose content
- **Celery.** Rich in potassium in your diet; has high water content
- **Cucumber.** Cool and refreshing; neutralizes the taste of vegetables with stronger flavors
- **Pineapples.** Contains bromelain, which can aid digestion
- **Apples.** Rich in antioxidants
- **Cabbage.** Rich in Vitamin C and folate; high water content
- **Beets.** Rich in beta-carotene, antioxidants such as lutein and zeaxanthin, calcium, and iron
- **Lemon.** Rich in Vitamin C; can neutralize acidity in the body

Apart from the abovementioned fruits and vegetables, Koff states that we can also add other "elements" into the mix to improve taste and nutritional value. Says Koff, "Freshly ground flax seeds, avocado, almond milk, coconut milk, tahini, or walnut oil could be tasty ways to add a little healthy fat to your juice."

Generally speaking, fruits and vegetables serve as excellent sources of a wide variety of various nutrients such as folate, potassium, vitamins and so on. With juicing, you can also help reduce, minimize or even completely avoid risks of various diseases such as cancers, type 2 diabetes, stroke, cardiovascular disease, and so on. Furthermore, vegetables rich in potassium can also help prevent bone loss and the formation of kidney stones.

Common Nutrients Found in Fruits

In relation to the list above, here are some more common nutrients found in fruits as analyzed by the US Department of Agriculture.

- **Enzymes.** Pineapples and papaya are two of the more popular fruits among those who drink extracted juice regularly. While they may be known for their taste, these are also beneficial for the enzymes they contain. Specifically, pineapples contain bromelain, while papayas contain papain. These enzymes aid digestion in the gastrointestinal tract.

- **Tartaric Acid.** This can strengthen the immune system; it can be found in fruits such as apples, apricots, pineapples, grapes, and avocados, as well as in sunflower seeds. Tartaric acid can also help achieve lowered levels of glucose and A1C levels, improved glucose tolerance, and improved intestinal absorption. It is also known for its antioxidative and antibacterial activities.

- **Citric Acid.** Commonly found in the family of citrus fruits, including limes, lemons, oranges and grapefruits, citric acid can also be found in other more popular fruits such as strawberries, pineapples, cranberries and peaches, to name a few. Citric acid has numerous benefits, such as preventing the formation of kidney stones, neutralizing free radicals that can lead to cancer, serving as an antioxidant, and so on.

- **Malic Acid.** Malic acid is found in apples, plums, apricots, cherries, grapes, lemons peaches, bananas, and prunes. Malic acid can aid digestion, initiate detoxification (particularly removing strontium and aluminum), support aerobic metabolic functions, and assist in energy production.

Fruits and Vegetables to Aid Weight Management

Perhaps one of the top reasons why juicing has become so popular these days is that many women want to manage their weight, lose a few pounds, and gain a leaner body. If you have the same reasons, then you made the right choice. Juicing has been proven to aid weight management.

In fact, The Centers for Disease Control and Prevention provides a list of fruits and vegetables, which they recommend as part of a healthy weight-loss diet routine. Below, let us take a look at some of the fruits and vegetables that have been proven to help people lose weight.

Spinach, according to The American Council on Exercise, is a prime example of a healthy food that should be included in your diet program. Spinach is a low-calorie but nutritious vegetable rich in iron, folate, magnesium, the powerful antioxidant known as Quercetin, as well as Vitamins A, C and K. People who love eating carbohydrate-rich fattening foods such as corn, rice or pasta, may substitute these with spinach, which only contains 7 calories per serving.

Watermelons are excellent fruits that you can include in your juicing program. Aside from their taste, they can help you lose weight because they are very filling while having low calories. In addition, the whitish portion of watermelon (the part between the skin and the red-colored flesh, is rich in citrulline, an amino acid commonly found in sports drinks to help decrease muscle fatigue. Thus, by drinking watermelon juice, you can exercise for longer periods.

Grapefruits only contain around 40 calories apiece. Based on a study published in the "Journal of Medicinal Food," compounds found in grapefruit improve your body's ability to control blood glucose levels. In terms of weight loss, it has been shown that eating half a piece of grapefruit prior to every meal may help you lose up to a pound a week.

Furthermore, grapefruits contain a compound that improves tissue sensitivity to insulin, which in turn, assists in fat loss. Finally, similar to watermelons, grapefruits are also very filling (with a water content of at least 90%).

Artichokes are excellent staples of a diet program because they can help curb the appetite, similar to other water-based fruits ad vegetables, without packing on the extra calories.

Fruits and Vegetables to Avoid

Although juice can be extracted from most fruits and vegetables, there are some that are considered "unjuiceable." These fruits and vegetables are probably best consumed whole or raw, rather than being juiced.

First in the list is the avocado, which turns oily, mushy and superosft fruit that yields little to no juice. As a new juicing devotee, maybe you should just stick to guacamoles for now.

Second is another obvious fruit, which is just as mushy as an avocado. We are talking about non-other than a banana. Because they have little water content, they are simply not ideal for juicing.

Third is the less popular winter squash—it is so tough, difficult to slice, and has little water content to yield a reasonable amount of extracted juice. The tough exterior may even damage less sturdy juicers, so it's best to stray from this vegetable altogether.

Fourth in the list are eggplants. Similar to a banana, an eggplant will not yield any reasonable amount of juice and will only turn super mushy and unusable when processed through a juicer.

Finally, we have rhubarbs. These have tough outer layers that can damage the slicers of centrifugal juicers or the blades of masticating or twin gear juicers. Beyond difficulty in preparation, rhubarbs also have high amounts of oxalic acid, which binds with the calcium in your body, rendering it useless.

Quick Shopping Tips

We have now basically presented an overview of what you should (should not) include in your shopping cart. Having gone through the previous sections of this chapter, you may have already created a list in mind as to what you should buy on your next shopping trip.

Now, let us give some important tips about shopping itself. As a novice fan of juicing, you may have or have not yet experience shopping for more produce in a conscious and selective manner. To help you survive this experience, here are a few shopping tips for you!

- **Tip#1.** It would be better if you make a detailed shopping list before you leave the house. This way, you can buy everything you need faster. As you make your list, you can go back to the early sections of this chapter so that you can identify what fruits and vegetables you want to try out first.

- **Tip#2.** As you make your list, it would also be ideal if you conduct a little online research as to what fruits and vegetables are in season. Buying in-season produce guarantees that you get them fresh and at a lower price.

- **Tip#3.** Remember the Dirty Dozen and the Clean Fifteen? Do keep these in mind as well while you are finalizing your shopping list. Remember, the Dirty Dozen are the produce that you should buy as organic produce while the Clena Fifteen are produce that are safe enough for consumption even if they are not organic.

- **Tip#4.** Do bring a recyclable shopping bag. This is way better than using plastic bags.

- **Tip#5.** Look for produce that has smooth, bruise-free skin. Whether you are buying organic or non-organic produce, anything that may have bruises or damage on the skin or the outerparts may indicate that it is no longer fresh or it has been mishandled.

- **Tip#6.** Do mind the price. Although you need more produce for your juicing needs, you don't have to buy everything in bulk. Moreover, check whether the price indicated is per unit or per kg. If the produce is priced according to weight, then only buy what you need. However, if the produce is priced per unit, then go buy the largest or heaviest one you can find.

- **Tip#7.** If you need to buy portions of, let's say, watermelons or green leafy vegetables, make sure that you buy those that have been bagged properly and surrounded by ice. You don't want to juice fruits or greens that are not fresh. Aside from bruising, you can also smell the produce as a quick way of checking freshness.

- **Tip#8.** Finally, ensure that the produce you have bought are packed and stored properly.

Juicing Mistakes and How to Avoid Them

Finally, you have already bought your juicer as well as selected and bought the fruits and vegetables you want to try. Before making your first glass of juice, we would like to leave you with a word of warning by listing down some common juicing mistakes.

Armed with such information, you can increase the likelihood that your first attempt will be a success. The success of your entire juicing program may ultimately rest on how good (or bad) your first glass of extracted juice tastes like and if your body accepts it well without adverse reaction.

To ensure success, here are some of the more common juicing mistakes and how you can avoid them.

Mistake #1 - Using too much sweeteners.

As we have explained earlier, while it is a good idea to start off with sweet, familiar-tasting fruits and vegetables, do avoid relying too much on these sweeteners. This is because too much sugar or fructose in your juice can feed harmful yeast and other organisms that can lead to excessive weight gain, fatigue, upset stomach, and so on.

Mistake #2 - Drinking juice on a full stomach.

Even some of the diehard juicers don't know this: extracted juice should only be taken with an empty stomach. The reason for this is pretty simple: drinking your juice on an empty stomach is the only way by which the nutrients, vitamins, and minerals will go straight to your bloodstream. If you forgot about it, you may want to wait two hours after eating a full meal before you can drink your juice.

Mistake #3 - Treating juice as a meal in itself.

This is a dangerous misconception about juicing. Juicing is only meant to supplement your regular food intake, and not replace it completely. Although extracted juice from fruits and vegetables are supercharged with nutrients, it cannot replace the other good stuff you can get from eating other kinds of food.

Mistake #4 - Not drinking the juice immediately after extraction.

Although juice can be stored for up to two days (only when you are using a high-end twin gear juicer), the best time to drink extracted juice is immediately after extraction. This is because the nutritional value becomes reduced the longer the juice sits. As we have mentioned earlier, fresh, extracted juice is best consumed within 20 minutes after extraction.

Furthermore, the extracted juice should be consumed at room temperature. This is because room temperature is the optimal temperature in which you can drink your juice. If you have prepared your juice beforehand, take out the container and let it stand for a few minutes before drinking it.

Mistake #5 - Not consuming juice properly.

It may sound surprising but did you know that you actually have to "chew" the juice before gulping it down. Here, "chewing" is not to be taken literally. In the world of juicing, "chewing" the juice means swishing the juice around in your mouth before gulping it down. The explanation for this is quite simple: as the juice mixes with your saliva, this process stimulates the digestion process, which is crucial to the body's ability to process the nutrients in the juice.

Mistake #6 - Using a dirty juicer.

For obvious reasons, it is a bad idea to use a dirty juicer in extracting a fresh glass if juice. For example, if you prepared juice in the morning, you need to clean your juicer thoroughly before using it again in the afternoon or in the evening. If you don't there may be issues with bacteria, buildup of debris within the small parts, and inefficiency of the juicer.

Mistake #7 - Using the same recipe over and over again.

Although you may eventually develop a preference for a certain combination of fruits and vegetables, it may be a bad idea to keep using that recipe over and over again. Aside from the obvious fact that your juice will taste blah if you keep using the same recipe, did you know that juicing the same green vegetables can actually lead to hormonal issues and build up of oxalic acid that may affect your thyroid gland. To avoid this, try experimenting on new blends. After all, variety is the spice of life!

In this chapter, we summarized specific nutrition-related information about fruits and vegetables that you can include in your shopping list. We also gave you a list of some popular produce, a few quick tips on how to combine them depending on what you want to achieve, and some information about shopping for produce.

Finally, we have also given you a list of common juicing mistakes that you must avoid at all costs. Armed with such information, you can now try juicing and hopefully continue with this program until you achieve the desired results.

Chapter 5. Juicing for Weight Loss

* * *

Another main reason why juicing has become the latest craze among health conscious people is weight loss. This is very true for women who want to maintain a healthy and sexy body amidst their very busy schedules. So, if you are a busy mother, career woman or both, you definitely don't have much time for weight loss or diet programs. But still, you look for ways to that can help you maintain your ideal weight and figure.

If you are a little overweight, you definitely want to lose weight by cutting down extra pounds on a weekly basis. You want these because you don't just want to have a healthy lifestyle. You want to have a gorgeous body because it makes you feel good and boosts your confidence and self-esteem. It also contributes in making your relationship with your husband spiced up.

However, most of the methods available today general consumes a lot of time. What you want is a solution that is very easy to do and does not consume so much time, right? For these, juicing might just be the right solution.

Before we proceed with the benefits of juicing for weight loss, we must define first what does "juicing" really means. These days, more and more people are now juicing for weight loss. But, does it really help in losing weight? Read on below to help you out.

In simplest terms, juicing refer to the process of extracting juice from fresh fruits and then, drinking it. Juicing can be also done with fresh vegetables. The best thing about it is that juicing only takes a few minutes and the juice is ready. With other meals, you need a lot of effort and time when it comes to preparation before you can even benefit from its nutrients. With juicing, however, you can enjoy complete nutrients enzymes, vitamins and minerals in almost an instant. It is also better as it does not require the digestive system to work hard. The body can fully and easily absorbs all the nutrients.

Benefits of Juicing

The next question is, is it more beneficial to consume extracted fruit or vegetable juice than to eat fresh and whole fruits and vegetables? The answer is a resounding yes. For one, the nutrients which go straight into our system make the body more efficient in performing its functions. Aside from this, there are also recent studies supporting the claim that juicing is healthier. Well, no one would find it difficult to agree with this. As we all know, the body needs to work when digesting the food that we eat. With juicing, the "work" that has to be performed when digesting foods can be used for other purposes.

Another great benefit of juicing is it allows our digestive system to have a break. This is important as the body can focus on other functions such as the healing process. That is why juicing is very helpful for people who are sick. They just have to juice the fruit or vegetable known to address a particular sickness. This is also very true when you have wounds or small cuts. The healing process is much faster if you include juicing as part of your medication. You can actually substitute juicing to over the counter medicines.

Another benefit, which women would surely love, is its crucial role in building metabolic processes. It also has a crucial role in the rebuilding and regenerating of healthy tissues that can make the body look more youthful.

Juicing also plays a significant role in various nutritional therapies. It is used in treating different illnesses and nutrient deficiencies. All in all, it has been proven that juicing is very effective in improving the well-being and overall health of an individual.

Juicing for Weight Loss

There is no denying that juicing has numerous benefits that have become crucial not just in treating nutrient deficiencies and in improving body processes but also in our busy schedules. With the possibility of making nutritious juices in an instant, many women can surely address the nutritional needs of their family. More than that, they can now also have an effortless way of maintaining a healthy and youthful body. But if you think that that is all juicing can offer, think again. Recently, it has been creating a buzz about its use for weight loss.

How can juicing aid in weight loss?

Anyone can surely lose weight by drinking fresh juice from fruits or vegetables as it helps in losing excess pounds. How does this happen? It aids in weight loss as it makes you calorie deficient. It brings about huge caloric deficiency because you only get to take in around 500 to 800 calories a day. So, the principle of juicing diet is achieving caloric scarcity by drinking juice on a daily basis. If you drink fresh juice daily, you can reduce calorie intake of up to 1,500 calories a day. This is equivalent to a weekly loss of about three pounds fat. The best thing about this diet is that it does not deprive you of energy. As a result, your metabolism will not crash and will help you realize an effortless and successful weight loss.

What's also great about drinking fresh juice is that it allows the body to absorb nutrients very easily. In this way, your body gets enough nourishment without having to take foods rich in carbohydrates and fats. This results to the easy flushing out of cholesterol. Another important thing is it does not create energy from the utilization of muscle tissues. With this, you can definitely maintain your sexy figure.

What are the benefits of juicing for weight loss?

Today, not everyone is already convinced about the effectiveness of juicing in losing weight. For example, the Center for Disease Control and Prevention has stated that there may be a connection between fresh fruit or vegetable juice intake and weight loss. However, they have also stated that fresh juice from fruits and vegetables have significantly low calories. It also makes you fell full after drinking, which helps you to avoid eating foods with higher calorie such as chips and chocolates.

With these, juicing has definitely become a popular way of losing weight nowadays. Consuming fresh fruit and vegetable juice has numerous advantages. Read on below to know more about these.

- **Fresh juice allows you to get all varieties of carbohydrates and complex vitamins.** This is practical as you don't have to worry about what kind of foods rich in carbohydrates to eat. It is also practical because you don't have to allot budget for other carbohydrates-rich foods.

- **You also get a lot of antioxidants which have numerous benefits as well.** AS you know, antioxidants are known to help lower the risk of developing diseases that are lifestyle-related. Examples of these are diabetes and heart disease. Moreover, antioxidants also help in preventing different types of cancer.

- **Fresh juice is the perfect alternative to your multivitamins pill.** You may not believe it but, yes, you can have fresh juice everyday and do away with your daily multivitamins intake. It is a perfect replacement as it is full of vitamins and minerals.

- **Drinking fresh juice also helps in cleansing your body.** In particular, it greatly helps in cleaning u your gut, which is essential in preventing colon cancer. It also helps in the proper function of the different internal organs.

- **You get all the benefits without any disadvantages or negative effects if you use organic fruits and vegetables.** With organic materials, you don't have to worry about pesticides and other harmful chemicals that huge agricultural crops companies use. As you know, chemicals that were taken by the body through consumption of foods can have a huge effect on the health of the individual. For women, it can affect the development of the fetus when they are pregnant.

- **If you want an excellent snack, nothing can be better than fresh juice.** For one, it gives you all the nutrients you need without leaving you overstuffed. Another advantage is that it can give your diet the variety it needs.

- **If you have hydration issues, drinking fresh juice can solve this.** Aside from the vitamins and minerals, fresh juice has water that can keep you hydrated.

- **You can achieve your objective of losing weight by drinking fresh fruit and vegetable juice as it has high phytonutrients.** These nutrients are essential in supporting your body to have greater balance. So, if your diet has high phytonutrients, you can definitely lose weight in the timeline you have set.

- **You can do away with your purely carbohydrate or meat protein diet.** With fresh juice, you can have a wider option in terms of vitamin choice.

- **You get the maximum nutritional value from fresh juice as you juice raw fruits and vegetables.** On the other hand, the commercial drinks contain a lot of preservatives which are known to cause negative side effects in your health. With this, fresh juice becomes more preferred than commercial juice by more and more health-conscious women.

- **The dissolved fiber helps in maintaining the level of cholesterol in our body.** AS you consume fresh juice, the fiber it contains gets dissolved in your intestines and bloodstream later on. This makes it perfect for individuals with cholesterol level problems.

- **Many think that fresh juice is not palatable.** Well, they are wrong. You can actually create more palatable and tasty fresh juice as you can create one using different fruits and vegetables. You can actually create your own juice recipe. Moreover, you can create a recipe that can very well address the nutrients your body is deficient of.

- **Fresh juice is cheaper and better.** This is because there are many wonderful and flavorsome recipes of fresh fruits and vegetables that you can try. With this, you can have so many options even if you are on a tight budget. We mothers will surely be happy about this as we always face the difficulty of budgeting money for house expenses.

- **A lot of mothers face the problem of their children lacking appetite during mornings.** As mothers we are always concerned about the health of our children. That is why we buy multivitamins that can help them have more appetite. With juicing, this can be addressed with spending money on multivitamins. Fresh juice can be a perfect breakfast for anyone and can greatly help in improving the appetite.

- **For people that really want to target the lowering of their cholesterol level, they can follow a juicing diet program with fruits and vegetables that target cholesterol.** Fresh juice is very effective as it has no saturated fats or added sodium.

- **Another great thing about juicing is that you can have fresh juice whenever you want.** This means that juicing is flexible with your time particularly with your very busy schedule. Career women would find it very helpful.

- **For people who have addiction to caffeine, carbohydrate, fat or alcohol, juicing is the solution.** Drinking of fresh juice can help them stay away from these addictions. As we know, being addicted to these unhealthy food elements is harmful to our health. These are the ones that cause diseases and cancer. BY treating addiction fat, alcohol and carbohydrate, one would really lose weight as a result. Mothers can train their children to drink fresh juices in their early years. In this way, the children would less likely develop addiction to unhealthy foods.

For the longest time, pineapples have been known to help in losing weight. That is why there are numerous companies, with canned pineapples and pineapple juice as products that invest in TV advertisements to promote the benefits of pineapple particularly in weight loss. To know if this is true, read on below to have more knowledge.

Pineapple for Weight Loss

In general, fruits and vegetables have relatively lower calories than other food items such as processed and canned foods. For example, a slice of pineapple only has 40 calories. This is very lower as compared to biscuits or cookies that have more than 100 calories. So, even if you consume 2 slices of pineapple you won't gain weight as it has low caloric content. Another reason why it helps in losing weight id that it has no protein or fat content. It contains Vitamin C, Manganese, fiber and a lot of antioxidants that help people maintain a healthy body.

The water and fiber will help in filling you up. With this, you would not want to look for other unhealthy foods as you are already full. Having weak bones is another problem that many women suffer from. The Manganese from pineapple can help in strengthening bones. Eating too much makes you feel bloated. This definitely contributes to gaining a lot of weight if not prevented. This can be addressed by the Pectin present in pineapples. If coupled with Vitamin C, it helps you prevent bloating. Another great thing about pineapples is it has Bromelain, which is also known to help prevent the onset or development of cellulite. Bromelain also helps in promoting muscle elasticity and muscle strength.

With all these, one may assume that pineapples really do help in weight loss. However, do pineapples have special properties that greatly promote in weight loss? The answer is no. It can help but it can't really promote weight loss. Pineapples won't help you burn fat, which is a crucial part of losing weight. It definitely won't help in burning fat because it can't keep your blood sugar at a low level. It has a glycemic index that is relatively higher than other fruits.

The glycemic index (GI) refers to a numerical scale that is used to indicate how high and fast a certain food can raise blood sugar or blood glucose level. If a food has low GI, it will raise our blood sugar level in moderation. On the other hand, if a food has a high GI it may prompt a high rise in our blood sugar level, which is usually above the optimal level. This is unhealthy or undesirable as high blood sugar level worsens our cholesterol level, which is a factor why people gain so much weight. With these, it should be clear by now that pineapples don't really promote weight loss. It can help, so it would still be beneficial to include it in your diet.

You can use pineapples to replace your usual foods that have higher caloric content. However, you have to take note that you need to eat fresh pineapples and not the canned ones. Canned pineapples are loaded with sugar, which makes it really unhealthy. It also has lesser nutrient content as most of the nutrients are lost during processing.

Banana for Weight Loss

Another fruit that many people believe to promote weight loss is banana. Unlike pineapples, bananas have higher caloric content. A regular size has 108 calories and around 17.5 grams of carbohydrates. With these, there is also a myth that bananas are not good in weight loss diet programs as it has high calories and carbohydrates. However, it has low glycemic index equal to 51. With this, one might certainly think that it is really helpful in losing weight.

Whether it promotes weight loss or not, there is no denying that bananas are among the most nutritious foods. For one, it is dense with minerals and vitamins. It is rich in potassium, which is important in the regulation of blood pressure. It is also high in fiber and low in fat. These are essential in helping you feel full for a longer time. If this is achieved, you won't feel the need to eat a lot or frequently. As a result, you would lose weight.

The craze about bananas as great weight loss food has become even more talked about when the Morning Banana diet was developed by Hitoshi Watanabe. It even became more popular when Japanese opera singer Kumiko Mori announced that she lost a significant amount of weight in pounds. According to her, she lost 15 pounds in just a few weeks. During that time, it was a phenomenal weight loss diet among Japanese people as it is said to be the easiest and fastest way of losing weight. It became known around the world through magazine articles, TV shows, and word of mouth. The Watanabes have also written a book about the diet.

However, all these don't still answer the question whether bananas promote weight loss or not. Well, the answer is no. Again, like pineapples, bananas don't help in the burning of fat. If fat is not burned, then you would not lose weight. However, it also helps in helping you lose weight if included in your diet program. Again, it does not promote but it can help in losing weight. According to food experts, bananas can help people lose weight if eaten in moderation. From this, it can be concluded that bananas don't really promote weight loss but can help if included in the diet program as snack.

Banana is a great food item as snack in your diet because it has potassium, which necessary in a low-calorie diet. A low-calorie diet with low potassium can lead to cardiovascular diseases, diarrhea, impaired cellular function and growth of muscles, and severe exhaustion. If you are planning to stick to a 1200-calorie diet, you can include a medium-sized banana. This will account for 9% of your total daily calorie intake. In this way, eating bananas helps you become successful in your goal of losing weight.

By this time, it should be very clear that pineapples and bananas don't promote weight loss. These fruits only help you in losing weight. What needs to be considered is the amount of calorie you have to take daily. From this, you will base the amount or size of pineapple and banana you have to eat everyday or for certain days of the week.

Skin, Hair and Nails – Beauty Anti Aging

Aside from weight loss, beauty is another primary reason why more and more people are drinking fresh juice from fruits and vegetables. In particular, a lot of women are now into juicing because of its anti-aging powers. When it comes to beauty, the skin, hair and nails are the first ones that we people see in a person. With this, we always adopt ways that can improve the health and glow of our skin, hair and nails.

Juicing for Healthy, Smooth and Glowing Skin

As women, we always want to stay beautiful. One way of achieving that is by having a glowing skin. Our skin glows if it is healthy from the inside. If we are following a healthy diet, it will reflect in the smoothness and glow of our skin. That is why many women are also patronizing skin care products. Millions of women use numerous skin products such as lotion, moisturizer, cream, body scrubs and many others. However, many of these products have chemicals that may affect our health. With this, there are now companies that create and produce organic skin care products. However again, this is just one part of nurturing and nourishing the skin. Our efforts to nurture it from the outside become incomplete if we don't eat the right and healthy foods.

In nourishing our skin through consumption of good food completes our goal of making our skin look healthy and youthful. That is why many of us include a lot of fruits and vegetables in our daily meals to ensure that we get all the vitamins, minerals and anti-oxidants needed for our skin's health. However, as busy mothers or career women, we don't usually have the time to prepare healthy meals. That is why many of us are looking for easier and more convenient alternatives to ensure that we and our family enjoy palatable and at the same time guilt-free meals.

When it comes to skin care, juicing has become the craze today as it allows us to get almost all of the nutrients that we need in just one glass of fresh juice from different fruits and vegetables. This has been the talk for so many women. But is juicing really helpful in taking care of your skin? Or it only worsens the condition? The answer is it depends on your diet program and how you treat juicing. To clear these issues, we can consider the case of Hollywood celebrity Jennifer Aniston who treats juicing as part of her normal consumption of meals. This means that she does not undergo pure juicing diet or never resorted to juicing diet at all. She still eats the regular meals she follows everyday and drinks fresh juice as part of her daily consumption.

On the other hand, many food experts say that the juicing diet does more harm than good. According to Dr. Sam Bunting, a cosmetic dermatologist, your skin will dry up if you follow a juicing diet. This is because your skin does not get the essential fatty acids it needs. Furthermore, he said that if your skin is always prone to dryness you may experience development of patches of eczema. This is because the barrier function of the skin is compromised if it does not get the enough amounts of essential fatty acids.

Sticking to pure juicing diet also has long term effects that would horrify you. Juicing diet is low in calorie and this makes the insulin levels to spike and crash. Initially, this causes break-outs. This insulin cycle alters the structures of elastin and collagen in the body over time. As a result, they become stiffer. This causes the skin to look prematurely old, which women never dream of. What we want is to maintain a youthful and glowing skin.

So, if you really want to get all the benefits of fresh juice from organic fruits and vegetables follow the recommendation of dietitian Natalie Jones. She said that it would be best if you have fresh juice as one of your five a day. She further said than consuming more than that won't do you any more good. It won't give you extra benefits but rather more harm.

Juicing for Healthy and Vibrant Hair

Aside from our skin, our hair is another part that we need to nurture and nourish. AS said it is our crowning glory and, thus, we have to ensure that it gets all the nutrients necessary for it to look shiny and silky. Today, there are also a lot of hair products that we patronize. Some of these are shampoo, hair conditioner, hot oil, hair dye, and others. Again, like commercial skin care products, these also have chemicals that may do harm to our hair later on in our life.

To address this, many are now also resorting to organic hair products. However, these products are usually more expensive than the commercial ones. With this, juicing seems to be the most effective and yet more affordable alternative. But like juicing for skin care, it may also do you more harm than good if you don't do the right thing. What then is the right thing to do? How should we treat juicing in so far as nourishing the hair is concerned?

If you do away with your normal five a day and replace it with more fresh juice, you may suffer from hair loss later on. If you think you are getting all the nutrients from fresh juice you wouldn't know how to explain it. According to Philip Kingsley, a renowned trichologist, you may experience hair fall two to three months after you start your juicing diet. He said that he had seen women coming to him with unexplained hair loss. But after some discussions, it turned out that there were following an extreme juicing diet.

According to him, hair loss happens when the body stops producing hair. If the body does not get all the nutrients it needs, it powers down or stops the processes that it considers not essential to life. One is the production of hair. With extreme juicing, or pure juicing diet, you definitely don't get to have all the nutrient, vitamins and minerals that your body needs for it to perform all the functions and processes well. For sure, you would not want to lose hair and get bald. As women, we should know these as we may have a different or misleading presumption for our hair loss. One possible that we may think is cancer symptoms when it is only about the harms of extreme juicing diet.

Now that we know these things, we can make juice recipes that will nourish our hair but without compromising other nutrients that the body needs. For example, we can have fresh juice made out of fruits and vegetables that are good for the hair, and drink it as part of our morning or afternoon snack.

Juicing for Healthy Nails

Though the skin is biggest and most recognizable part of our body, the nails also reflect our health. We are not getting all the nutrients that our body needs if our nails look dull, brittle and has some white spots. This means that we are lacking certain vitamins and minerals. There are many ways by which this can be addressed. One way is through the use of nails products like nail polish. However, this is just like a band aid solution as it does not really address the nutrient deficiency of our body.

One great way to have healthy nails is to adopt juicing. It is more practical than purchasing nail products. Your nails can look their best if you let them breathe. So, it can only breathe if you stop using nail polish. It should not be hard for you to let go of nail cosmetics a you can save money from it. Your nails will also look their best if you drink fresh juice using certain fruits and vegetables known to provide nourishment to your nails. Drinking fresh juice allows your nails to grow beautifully and stay strong.

To be effective in nourishing your nails, you have to consider nutrients and vitamins that are necessary in making your nails completely bioavailable. This means that you are effective in the assimilation of all the nutrients from the juice you consume. So, you need to consider fruits and vegetables that are rich in Biotin, Zinc, Vitamin C and Omega 3 fatty acids. However, if you just eat these foods it would be a little harder for the nutrients to get into your bloodstream. But if you get these nutrients through juicing, it becomes easier for them to directly get into your bloodstream.

For your nails, you can use carrots, bananas, ginger, nuts, broccoli and leafy green varieties to create your juice. Combinations of these fruits and vegetables can give your skin the nutrients it needs such as Vitamin C and essential fatty acids. For example, if you want a juice high in Vitamin C, you can combine lemons, apples, ginger root and lime. If you want a juice rich in Omega 3 fatty acids, Biotin and Zinc, you can use pears, spinach and walnuts. Depending on what your nails need, there are specific fruits and vegetables that you have to combine. There are also juice recipes that you can follow if you want to achieve certain goals like longer and stronger nails. For this, you can use kale leaves without the stem, apricots with pits removed, mangoes, handfuls of blueberries, chia seeds, and green or red grapes.

Juicing for Beauty and Anti-Aging Purposes

There is no denying, fresh juice from fruits and vegetables can really make you beautiful and more youthful. With these, you might want to know what are some of the fruit and vegetables that you always have to keep in your refrigerator. Some of these are carrots, cucumbers and strawberries.

Carrots should always be present in your kitchen as it is rich in Vitamin C, which helps in promoting healthy eyesight. It also has antioxidants which help in boosting the immune system. This is essential especially nowadays that there are a lot of viruses and bacteria that may easily cause our sickness. Carrots taste really good when you combine them with apples.

Cucumbers also contain Vitamin C. It has potassium and iron. It is highly recommended for women who want to flush out heavy toxins from their bodies through gentle detoxification. This is because the cucumber is a mild diuretic and is mostly made up of water. These promote frequent urination which is a way of flushing out toxins from your body.

Strawberries, unlike vegetables such as spinach, are more likeable. A strawberry is also high in Vitamin C, which helps in maintaining a strong immune system. It is also known to have antioxidants that fight free radicals. For people who suffer from arthritis, strawberries are good for them as these are anti-inflammatory. Lastly, strawberries are essential in maintaining strong and healthy connective tissues such as bones and skins.

With the wonders of fresh juice from fruits and vegetables, women can now have a more affordable, healthier, safer and more enjoyable way of caring for their skin, hair and nails. They can now live without the commercially produced cosmetic products which have a lot of chemicals and preservatives. Juicing is definitely a lot better as it nourishes your skin, hair and nails from the inside. If you are well fed with the nutrients you need, it will reflect on the outside. You don't have to use band aid solutions anymore. You just have to remember that you can optimize juicing to your advantage if you use organic produce and if you include juicing as one of your five a day. You can even improve your youthful look by applying organic beauty products on your skin, hair and nails.

Chapter 6. Juicing for Vitality

* * *

We all have to admit it—life will not be complete without a bit of groove. No matter how busy you are, having some spice in your life, and some hot and exciting nights (or even days) do make a (huge) difference on how your mood and overall outlook in life goes. Even the busiest fulltime mom or the most career-committed professional needs this. Otherwise, you can prepare to be called Cruella De Ville in the future or simply feel empty until you die. But that would be the worst-case scenario here. This is exactly why we are talking about simple yet effective ways to revive that sexual vitality—how to get your groove back with juicing.

Unlike what is commonly known to many, lovemaking is both a biological need and a gift that enables us to express our love with another human being. It allows us to connect with our partners. It is considered as the most powerful demonstration of our existence as human beings.

However, women are often subject to sexual deprivation because of their social status— normally seen as superheroes capable of doing numerous roles (such as being a wife, a mom, a worker, a driver to the kids, a teacher, a caregiver to all sick patients in the household, and a janitor!) all at the same time.

The sexual benefits of juicing have become quite popular in the United States and in other countries as well. The reason behind such fact is that more and more women are now showing some kind of sexual inability and lose their libido at a very early age. In the US, about 43% of all women suffer from such dysfunction—each one attributing their condition to various reasons. But before we discuss how juicing helps you revive your zest for sex, let us first discuss why your libido may be going down for quite some time.

Stress

The most common cause of sexual dysfunction is stress. The latter basically keeps your mind and body tired, unable to function at its most capable extent, turn your energy levels down, and leaves you out of time for love and other things aside from your career (or your household chores). This is why some people say that sex and satisfaction is just for men—married men, that is. While women, who are tied to taking care of their children, or career women who are focused on excelling and succeeding among others, often lose their desire for orgasm and all the good things that come before that.

The human body has its limits and once these are reached, other tasks are not fulfilled. Stress and over fatigue comes from too much work—whether at home or not. Women are generally turned on and become sexually excited through mental and emotional means. Unlike men who are visually aroused in general, women need some sort of sensual foreplay to get aroused. If they are mentally and emotionally stressed, the physical stage of getting excited for sex is blocked. Stressed women find it more difficult to reach orgasm when they are exhausted. This is because stress weakens the brains ability to send signals to the body, and therefore impairs our endocrine glands to do their work.

Aside from having the right juicing diet, you must learn to de-stress and unwind. Conscious efforts to reduce factors that add to your stress levels will definitely contribute to having more vitality in life. Make sure to have breaks every once in a while, go on vacations, listen to relaxing music, or simply take time to lay down in bed and have enough rest from your daily routine. There are a lot of stress reduction programs and techniques that you can use to make your juicing work at its fullest capacity.

Unhealthy Lifestyle

Having an unhealthy lifestyle does not only affect your overall well-being. It largely affects your vitality and how good you do in bed. Do not wonder if you keep trying to get that groove back but are having a hard time getting full pleasure after having rounds of beer. Everyone, whether male or female, become less active in bed after getting some booze.

Alcohol naturally impairs our senses and thus affects our ability to participate in sexual activities and lowers down the production of testosterone, a hormone needed to boost your libido to its normal level.

It is true that taking red wine regularly in limited and planned amounts is healthy for women who need to relax. However, taking more than two glasses will have negative effects on your sexual performance, and should be avoided if you want to have some romantic nights with your partner.

Likewise, the intake of too much caffeine (whether from coffee, tea, chocolate, etc.) interjects with the production of hormones, and in fact interferes with women's menstrual cycles. This means that your libido is also affected by excessive drinking of coffee. If you are addicted to any of these caffeine-rich and addictive drinks, you might as well limit your intake. Otherwise, juicing might not just work for you.

While chocolates can act as aphrodisiacs for men, women who want to get some vitality up should avoid taking too much of these sweets.

Another factor that largely contributes to an unhealthy lifestyle that may affect your libido is smoking. Aside from the unwanted smell that it may cause your breath, smoking can be an overall killer for your love life. Because of the numerous toxins found in tobacco smoke, your body's oxygen will dramatically decrease and may cause blood vessel damage, and therefore decreases blood flow. Good blood circulation is vital in arousal, and contributes to the pleasure that you get from making love. So it is just right to say that anyone who needs some groovy nights should eliminate bad habits such as smoking, where lead, nicotine, cadmium, carbon monoxide, benzopyrene and a lot of other toxic chemicals take its toll through the most unwanted diseases such as cancer. Having illnesses such as cancer and losing your vitality would be the last thing you would want to happen to your busy life.
Aside from toxins you can get from smoking, people from all over the world today suffer from artificial food ingredients and chemicals that likewise inhibit good blood circulation, and lessen your energy for life's most exciting details. Preservatives, additives, artificial flavorings, coloring, and pesticides are big culprits for the human race's dwindling state of health. These chemicals bombard our bodies and take the place of the necessary nutrients that we need in order to perform well—at work or in bed.

Not having enough sleep also brings your energy levels down, and obviously takes you out of the mood for love (or anything else other than sleep, that is!). It is vital to know that even if you have the most helpful juicing diet, the lack of sleep will still haunt you and keep you out of your groove.

Hormonal Imbalance and Changes

Hormonal changes and imbalances caused by stress, biological impairments, or natural life events such as menstrual cycles, postpartum phases, and menopause, similarly affect your libido. Hormonal imbalances often trigger physical discomfort, most commonly characterized by mood swings, insomnia, hot flashes, digestive problems, and weight gain. When a woman nears her menstrual period, or has just given birth or undergone abortion, hormonal levels change drastically. The physical byproducts directly affect her gusto for romance and lovemaking. Nonetheless, hormonal imbalances brought about by menstruation, postpartum phases, and abortion naturally settle down unless you are in need of some medical attention. Once your hormones get back to their normal levels, the physical challenges will also go away and leave you more comfortable doing anything—and give you back your groove.

Libido is attributed to testosterone—the life force hormone that gets us going on and on in bed. Having low testosterone levels is equivalent to low libido. The roots of low testosterone levels may be stress, or medical conditions that cause their ovaries to function abnormally.

Now that you know the reasons for having low sexual vitality, the next thing to do is to see if you are one of the majority of women who suffer from loss of sexual appetite. This is crucial information that will help you seek the best juicing recipes apt for your particular condition.

Are You Losing Your Vitality?

There is more to juicing than a fit and healthy body. With the correct combination of your most favorite vegetables, fruits, and herbs that make up perfect recipes, you can even revive your sexual vitality without having to take synthetic medicine. There are a few things you can check to see if you are indeed losing your vitality.

The first thing you should ask yourself is "Am I significantly, but unexplainably losing my appetite for sex?". To answer this question, you can take note of the frequency of your initiative or your partner's granted initiatives to have sex. Low libido is demonstrated by indifference, the inability to perk up for sex. Women are opposite to men—as we grow older, our sex drive naturally stays longer because of increasing testosterone production. Males, as they get older, little by little lose their stride in bed because their production of testosterone decreases. This means that as you age, you must consider checking on your vitality, and see if it coincides with this fact.

Lesser libido also means taking more time before reaching orgasm, or having less pleasurable orgasms than before. Yes, orgasms differ at one time or another. The intensity of that blissful moment where you feel all your muscles contracting can be discerned and that is a factor you must consider. You may still be having sex in as frequent as you used to do, but the climax and the pleasure is another thing to look after. Sex is not just a routine—it is human's greatest gift of expression and should therefore serve its purpose: to make you feel love and loved in return. Sex without orgasm is just like doing your household chores or work assignments—it will only leave you exhausted and unfulfilled at the end of the day. So if you are often faced with exhaustion after having sex, you might be losing your groove unconsciously.

A lot of women suffer from the abovementioned factors due to loss of vaginal lubrication. The latter likewise shows they need more groove back.

If you are experiencing any of these, there is indeed a great need for you to focus on the right juicing recipes that will help you get your vitality return to its normal phase.

Juicing for Vitality

A lot of women, as they age, have less and less sex due to many reasons. Some women do not have sex at all. And what's the reason behind this? Generally, they lose their interest in lovemaking or they simply do not make time for it. Women who are at their 40's and beyond go through menopause, which some consider the end of sexual pleasure. However, contrary to this common misconception, menopause is actually another exciting stage in a woman's life wherein having sex no longer leaves you worried of getting an unplanned pregnancy. Then again, the hormonal imbalance it causes makes it a bit hard for women to enjoy this supposedly stimulating stage.

There are a lot of juicing recipes and suggested ingredients that are particularly advised for women who suffer from hormonal imbalance and loss of sexual vitality thereafter. A combination of beet, carrot, and ginger, with a hint of grape juice, helps bring back your hormonal levels to normal.

Squash, when juiced, adds to your body's production of the right hormones that will take your sexual desires up. Add a bit of cinnamon regularly to your daily dose of juice and you can expect to be ready for sex anytime.

There is a huge difference between aphrodisiacs and juicing for sexual vitality. The latter revives your energy and gives you most oomph in bed. Aphrodisiacs, on the other hand, simply makes you go hot and do not necessarily keep you in the groove. It is just to say that they will not make your orgasms more intense and the whole sexual experience more pleasurable.

Seeds and nuts, like sesame, sunflower, pumpkin seeds, chia, and hemp are best juiced with fruits. Beans and grains are likewise best for those who want to add vitality to their lives. Adding a bit of garlic, ginger, and cardamom gives a little flavor to your recipe, and likewise warms up your body as you would need it for some hot and romantic nights.

To help your blood circulate, make your body ready for complete and necessary arousal for a good sexual intercourse, turmeric, cayenne, and lemon will be the perfect addition to your juicing recipe. Regular intake of these healthy ingredients will help your blood circulate throughout your body, including your vagina and everything that surrounds it. Opposite to what we commonly believe, males are not alone in the need for excellent blood circulation to pump up their penis during lovemaking.

It also helps to include acai, berried, cruciferous vegetables, and mangosteen to your daily dose of healthy juicing recipes to promote a healthy liver. In return, your liver does its job in your body's blood circulation.

Here is an example of a juicing recipe for women in search of good vitality:

Prepare 4 carrots. Make sure to leave it half-peeled as the skin is the healthiest part of this root. Add 2 stalks of celery. Celeries are rich in androsterone, a hormone that helps stimulates your sex drive. Add in 3 kale leaves and half a cucumber that will increase your libido and stamina. Use one knuckle of ginger to remove toxins in your blood and promote good blood circulation.

Another juicing recipe that will help bring your groove back:

Ingredients:

1. 1 large bulb of fennel (make sure to remove fronds and trim it)
2. 2" ginger knob
3. 3 ripe pears (best to choose organic ones to avoid unwanted chemicals and toxins)
4. 1 large bunch of watercress

5. 1 lemon

Cut the fennel bulb and pears into four parts. Peel and remove the pith from the lemon. Slice it in half. Place everything inside a juicer. Drink immediately to avoid separation of parts.

Juicing recipes are not hard to prepare. They involve a bit of slicing, paring, and peeling, and all you have to do is use a juicer to create than wonderful drink that will bring you vitality.

Here are other juicing recipe suggestions for a more active sex life:

Combine 4 kale leaves, half a cup of mango, 5 romaine leaves, half a cup of pineapple, half a cup of parsley sprigs, and half an inch slice of ginger. This powerful combination gives you a green smoothie that will bring your energy in bed back in no time. It is overall detoxifying, and helps boost blood circulation for an ultimate climax.

You can also try juicing 1 apple, half a cup of parsley or spinach, 4 unpeeled carrots, and 1 pared kiwi. This recipe is an energizer that will give you more drive as you feel your youthfulness once again.

A glass of pomegranate juice each day also brings your testosterone levels up, and therefore makes you yearn for sex—that is, the satisfying one.

The key to making an effective and enjoyable vitality juice that will bring your groove back is to know the basic ingredients (vegetables, fruits, nuts, roots, and the like) that basically promote good blood circulation, relaxation, more energy, better health and mood.

On the other hand, your efforts in juicing for vitality may reach its full potential in bringing back your sex appetite if you are not wary of the kind of food that you eat. As said in the previous chapters, it is crucial to choose your food if you are serious in practicing a healthy lifestyle, not to mention trying to regain your sexual vitality.

The following foods are a no-no for women who want to real and effective juicing for a more healthy and satisfying sex life:

1. **Fried food.** Trans fats that come from fried food—whether fruits, vegetables, or whatever—lower libido levels by clogging your blood vessels and veins and therefore giving your blood a hard time to circulate all throughout your body.

The effect? Your senses do not get as sensitive as they should, your sexual organs have lower reaction capabilities to romance stimulus, and all in all you lose your passion for sex and orgasm.

If you prefer to somehow eat your regular meals other than juicing, make sure to use healthy and proper cooking procedures that do not use oil, chemicals, or other toxins that will ruin your juicing diet. Try steaming or boiling your food to avoid unwanted fats.

2. **Soy products.** Soy products, although were believed to be of good benefit to people's health, have been found to promote higher levels of estrogen. In various studies done all over the world, people have proven that soy is one of the culprits for hormonal imbalance and takes away women's sex drive. A little amount should be okay, but daily big doses will mean a lot of negative effects on your body, including but not limited to sexual impotence and loss of interest.

3. **High fat dairy.** This can be found in cheese, ice cream, and milkshake which can aggravate pre-menstrual cycle syndromes and dysmenorrhea. Worst, high dairy fat can lower down your libido as well.

4. **Combination of flour and sugar.** Yes, you read that right. Anything that is made out of combined flour and sugar is a no-no. It combats our genuine objective to increase our vitality and get our groove back. Cupcakes, cakes, cookies, macaroons, muffins, brownies, and the like amplifies our glucose levels, and in turn causes hormonal imbalance and decreases our appetite for sex and romance.

Make sure to balance your diet and stick with those that can help boost your vitality. Juicing is an effective way to bring your groove back, but without the proper diet and exercise, you cannot expect to get the best results. Similarly, it is crucial to have a balanced and healthy lifestyle that enables your body to recuperate from all the hassles of being a superwoman, and gives you the space and time to care for yourself. Remember, reviving your appetite and energy for sex is affected by physical, mental, and emotional conditions.

Once you have managed to renew your lifestyle to a healthier one, change your diet to fit your juicing recipes, and maintained your intake of vitality juices, your love life will give you the best and most romantic love making experience—something you can call a reward for living such a healthy life.

Chapter 7. Juicing for Improved Health

* * *

Aside from the many simple yet tremendous things juicing brings to busy and career-focused women (and fulltime wives and moms), this remarkable technique to having a healthy lifestyle is an effective way to prevent cancer, diabetes, and digestive problems. Juicing, when done correctly, will improve your health, your overall outlook in life, your sex life, your abilities—basically your life. We are not trying to overvalue here. It is simply true that when your body ingests more nutrients and fiber, it is able to function well—better than that which intakes a lot of chemicals, meat, and all those unhealthy diet being promoted by big fast food chains and pricey restaurants.

The biggest question to most people who are new to juicing: What exact difference does it have compared to eating fruits and vegetables as a whole?

Vegetarians and vegans basically stick with the same ingredients as what juicing uses. Overall, eating vegetables and fruits as your main diet, combined with good sources of protein such as beans, nuts, and seeds, gives your body a complete set of nutrients that is needed for it to function well. To start giving you an idea of the health benefits of juicing, here is a detailed elucidation of what vegetables and fruits fundamentally provide our bodies.

Knowing the health benefits: Introduction to vitamins and minerals from veggies and fruits

Vitamin A is essential in the reproduction of cells, and helps build strong immunity against diseases. Some hormones are produced sufficiently with the support of this nutrient. It also promotes good eyesight, bone and teeth development, and contributes to how your hair and skin shines and glows. Vitamin A is found in vegetables like Bok Choy, Amaranth Leaves, Butternut, Broccoli, Chinese Broccoli, Squash, Carrots, Leeks, Kale, spinach, pumpkin, sweet potato, and cabbage. Fruits such as grapefruit, papaya, mango, cantaloupes, guava, watermelon, and tomatoes are a good source of Vitamin A.

Vitamin B1, also called thiamine, boosts your energy and therefore makes you go through your day despite your hectic schedule. It is fundamental in converting carbohydrates into useful energy. Most importantly, it promotes full function for the nervous system, the heart, and muscles. Thiamine deficiency leads to fatigue and weakness. This powerful vitamin can be found in vegetables such as spirulina, asparagus, butternut, corn, lima beans, peas, parsnips, sweet potato, Brussels sprouts, French beans, and okra. Fruits rich in thiamine are boysenberries, avocado, dates, guava, breadfruit, grapes, mango, loganberries, cherimoya, pineapple, watermelon, pomegranate, and grapefruit.

Riboflavin, otherwise known as vitamin B2, is an essential factor for normal body growth. It is likewise important in reproducing red cells. Like thiamine, it helps release energy from carbohydrates. Vegetables rich in riboflavin are artichoke, amaranth leaves, Brussels sprouts, asparagus, lima beans, mushrooms, bok choy, chineses broccoli, peas, sweet potato, peas, and swiss chard. Fruits that give you riboflavin are banana, avocado, dates, passion fruit, cherimoya, grapes, pomegranate, lychee, mulberries, prickly pear, and mangoes.

Vitamin B3 is another essential vitamin that the body gets from different foods. It is also called niacin, and it promotes a healthy digestive system. It also helps the skin and nerves to function. Like the previous two, niacin assists in converting carbohydrates to useful energy. Parsnips, spirulina, okra, artichoke, butternut, corn, squash, and peas are just a few of the many vegetables that provide us with this vitamin. Fruits such as boysenberries, dates, avocado, passion fruit, nectarine, peaches, and guava are among those which contain niacin.

Pantothenic acid or vitamin B5 helps produce hormones and good cholesterol which are vital in maintaining a healthy body. It is found in broccoli, squash, butternut, okra, mushrooms, corn, French beans, among others. Black currants, avocado, gooseberries, dates, cherimoya, raspberries, watermelon, starfruit, grapefruits, and breadfruit are also good sources of vitamin B5.

The same vegetables are also rich in vitamin B6, which contributes in creating antibodies for your immune system. Also called pyridoxine, this vitamin has a big role in processing protein intake. For people who have big intakes of protein, bigger amounts of pyridoxine is likewise needed. Otherwise, the person will suffer from convulsions, dizziness, confusion, and nausea.

Vitamin B9, which is found in most fruits and vegetables mentioned above, is essential in producing red blood cells and the nervous system. Women who plan to become pregnant should have sufficient intake of vitamin B9, which comes in the form of folate and folic acid.

Vitamin C is another essential vitamin that the body needs in order to have full function. It acts as an antioxidant that protects human cells from the bad effects of free radicals. It is also a good antiviral agent that blocks viral diseases. Amaranth leaves, broccoli, bok choy, butternut, squash, kale, green pepper, and swiss chard are vegetables with vitamin C. Fruits rich in vitamin C are strawberries, pineapples, mulberries, black currants, grapefruits, breadfruits, lychee, oranges, mangoes, kiwi, papaya, and passion fruit.

Vitamin E is another antioxidant that protects our bodies from oxidation damages. It also plays a significant role in the creation of red blood cells. It is vital and indispensable in putting vitamin K into use. Vitamin E is used by women to reduce scars and wrinkles, as it can heal broken skin tissues. This particular vitamin is found in a lot of fruits (i.e. blackberries, guava, avocado, black currants, breadfruit, blueberries, cranberries, boysenberries, loganberries, kiwi, papaya, mango, nectarine, mulberries, peaches, pomegranate, peach, and raspberries.

Most of the abovementioned vegetables and fruits likewise contain vitamin K, which has an important part in blood clotting. This vitamin is essential in regulating calcium levels in the blood, and activates proteins that add to maintaining healthy bones. Chinese pears, plums, tomatoes, alfalfa sprouts, cauliflower, celery, cucumber, and rapini are a few more vegetables that provide vitamin K to our bodies.

Vitamin D maintains our calcium and phosphorus levels in the blood. It helps the body absorb calcium and magnesium, and therefore promotes good and healthy bone and teeth development. Mushrooms are the only vegetables (or non-meat product, rather) that contains vitamin D.

On the down side, Vitamin B12, which plays an important role in your body's metabolism, cannot be found in vegetables and fruits. Fish, meat, poultry, and dairy products are the only food that act as sources of vitamin B12.

Vegetables and fruits are also rich in essential minerals that the body needs. We have already mentioned how calcium and magnesium play and important role in bone development. Calcium likewise lessens insomnia and promotes the correct contraction of muscles, clotting of blood, and efficient functioning of the nerves.

Copper helps the body absorb and use iron, and thus contributes to the formation of red blood cells. Consequently, it promotes good supply of oxygen to the body, which in turn allows for better nutrient absorption.

Iron, which comes from most fruits, is especially found in raisins. Manganese, Phosphorus, Potassium, Selenium, Sodium, and Zinc are other minerals found in most vegetables.

Now that you are familiar with all the vitamins and minerals that can be found in vegetables and fruits, let us answer the first question that was asked earlier in this chapter. What exact difference does it have compared to eating fruits and vegetables as a whole?

Benefits of Juicing

Juicing, unlike eating your vegetables and fruits in whole, makes it easier for the body to absorb all the nutrients in them. A lot of people suffer from digestive problems, and juicing somehow digest the food for them. Instead of worrying what type of food will be easier for them to digest, they will now have to pay attention to the vitamins and minerals that they need in order to maintain a healthy diet.

Today's fast food filled world suggest more meat and artificial diets rather than eating healthy, fresh, and chemical free. Children are brought up at McDonald's, literally spend their birthdays there, and are trained to love unhealthy foods over healthy vegetables. This makes it very difficult for them to eat vegetables despite the need for it. If you are one of those who were overshadowed by the McDonald dream, juicing can be a huge help for you to start taking more veggies without the torment. One glass of vegetable juice may be sufficient to supply your body with enough vitamins and minerals that you need—given that you are able to combine the right ingredients as you add juicing to your diet.

Juicing is a fun way to enhance your diet and give your body an overall boost from stress and illnesses. You can add different flavors to your not-so-loved vegetables to make them taste more palatable, or do an experiment on your favorite fruits.

Juicing Against Cancer

Cancer is one of the greatest fears of Americans when it comes to their health. It is one of the most common causes of death, and is still rising at present. There are many things that contribute to why cases of cancer are increasing. Generally, cancer is caused by different factors including genetics, chemicals from smoking tobacco, unhealthy diet and abnormal physical activities, overexposure to the sun's UV rays, exposure to radiation, and other carcinogens.

Some families genetically pass on cancer from one generation to another. However, this does not necessarily mean that all families with cancer patients from different generations have hereditary cancer. Different generations in a family with multiple cancer patients often inherit other types of disease that increase the risk of cancer. In reality, cancer itself cannot be inherited. People inherit abnormal genes that may lead to certain types of cancer. This constitutes only 5-10% of all cancers.

This being said, we can easily state that even 'inherited' cancer can be prevented by following a healthy diet and lifestyle. This is contrary to popular belief that 'inherited' cancer is inevitable.

Cigarette smoking is identified as the "major single cause of cancer mortality [death] in the United States", according to the 1982 report from the United States Surgeon General. 16.5% of adult women smoke cigarettes—the same culprit for 30% of all deaths caused by cancer. 87% of the deaths among lung cancer patients is caused by smoking. Second hand smoke is also a cause of cancer. Although there is still a need for further studies and evidences, second hand smoke has been seen to cause breast cancer among women.

Likewise, smoking is strongly attributed to lung cancer, oral cavity cancers, larynx cancer, esophagus and pharynx cancers, stomach, pancreas, cervix, kidney, bladder, ovarian, colorectum cancers, and acute myeloid leukemia.

The most common type of cancer in women in the US is breast cancer. However, the most common cause of cancer death among women is still lung cancer. Causes of breast cancer vary as well—from aging, genetics, history of breast cancer, breast lumps, exposure to estrogen, obesity, exposure to radiation and carcinogens, and implants. To prevent breast cancer, a good and healthy lifestyle should be developed. It has also been learned that breast cancer survivors are more likely to have diabetes.

Fortunately, there are many vegetables and fruits that contain nutrients that act as antioxidants and prevent cancer. Carrot juice helps in detoxifying the body, particularly the liver, and helps flush out excess fat and unwanted chemicals (those that you get from eating genetically modified products, artificial flavorings and additives). As your liver functions to its full capacity, your fats are easily burned and thus keeps you away from being overweight. Prevention of the latter contributes in preventing different types of cancer. Beets add more detoxifying agents to your body and further pushes toxic chemicals out of your body. Drinking beet juice in large amounts is known to terminate cancers and tumors in the body.

Cabbage, which is rich in vitamins and minerals, is also a good choice to combine with carrot juice. As long as it is pesticide-free, cabbages consumed regularly help in preventing cancer just as studies show.

Green leafy vegetables are high sources of antioxidants, and promote the formation of red blood cells. Most green and leafy vegetables contain almost all essential vitamins and minerals, so juicing them will be perfect for those who want to make sure their bodies are fully maintained.

Juicing Against Diabetes

Diabetes is an illness that is demonstrated by a complex of different diseases like hyperglycemia. Diabetes happens when your body does not produce enough insulin that will help your body absorb and transform glucose into energy. Insulin comes from the pancreas.

There are two types of diabetes—type 1 and type 2 diabetes. Type 1 diabetes is caused by the inability of the pancreas to produce insulin because its beta cells are destructed by the body's immune system. This happens when there is an autoimmune deficiency. Although type 1 diabetes is not caused by a virus, experts suggest they are closely link to each other.
On the other hand, type 2 diabetes is the most common type of diabetes among US and non-US citizens. It is caused by multiple factors, which is worsened by the body's inability to efficiently make use of insulin. The most overpowering factor is having a family history of this kind of illness. Obesity, an inactive lifestyle, aging, and unhealthy diet contribute to the risk of having type 2 diabetes. Other illnesses such as pancreatitis or pancreatectomy, glucagonoma, polycystic ovary syndrome, and steroid induced diabetes also potential causes of type 2 diabetes.

In the US, more than 12.6 million women aged 20 years and beyond suffer from diabetes. 68% of diabetics (who are 65 years old and above) have heart disease. 67% of people with diabetes who are 20 years old and above have high blood pressure. As much as 70% of diabetics suffer from different forms of nervous system injury. In 2007, diabetes was found to have played a role in the death of more than 231,000 deaths.

Good thing there is a wide array of juicing recipes especially prepared for diabetics. Since diabetes is a complex group of diseases characterized with insufficient production of insulin or ineffective use of insulin (or both) causing hyperglycemia, there are a lot of vegetables and juices you can use to prevent risk factors from developing. A lot of vegetables and fruits are beneficial to diabetics as they help the body respond to insulin better, and give type 2 diabetics an easier way to trim down their bodies.

The basics of juicing for diabetics should begin with knowing what you need to avoid: glucose, sucrose, and fructose. Glucose is basically the type of sugar that comes from carbohydrates when broken down by the human body. Fructose is naturally found in fruits. Glucose and fructose is sucrose when combined.

To avoid sucrose, it is wiser for diabetics to stick with a vegetable juicing diet. However, one of the disadvantages of juicing is that it does not give as much fiber as eating whole vegetables do. Then again, by choosing the right vegetables that do not contain much carbohydrates, you will be able to stay away from complications and take advantage of the positive effects of juicing. Other people choose not to peel their vegetables so they can still get enough fiber that is very effective in regulating blood sugar.

Juicing recipes for diabetics are made up of non-starchy veggies which have small amounts of carbohydrates and contain a low glycemic index. However, studies show that processing food increases its glycemic index. This means that vegetable juice will probably contain a higher glycemic index compared to vegetables when eaten as a whole.

Asparagus is known to help keep sugar levels down. The intake of tomatoes, cucumber, Brussels sprouts, and cucumber contributes to the management of diabetes. Vegetables rich in manganese are good in keeping insulin resistance down. Vitamin C is an effective tool to prevent diabetes, and can be found in broccoli.

Cinnamon is likewise known to help in lowering resistance to insulin, and therefore promotes better insulin sensitivity. Adding cinnamon to your vegetable juice does not only have the positive effects to your body, but is easy to find, and incorporate to recipes, and adds a twist to boring juices.

Green leafy vegetables like spinach, kale, and collards are among the most nutritious and diabetic-friendly foods that you can use in your juicing recipe against diabetes. A combination of carrots, cucumber, spinach, celery, and a small slice of green apple works for those who need some nutrient boost without taking too much glucose and fructose.

Tomatoes can be combined with green pepper, ginger, celery, and garlic. You can also try to juice romaine lettuce with celery and tomatoes. Asparagus, carrots, and zucchini are also a perfect match to tomato juice.

Juicing Against Digestive Problems

Digestive problems are very common in Americans, which can be attributed to the growing unhealthy lifestyle in the country. There are many forms of digestive problems, ranging from short-lived reflux, to peptic ulcers, gallstones, chronic constipation, abdominal wall hernia, diverticular disease, gastrointestinal infections, inflammatory bowel disease, irritable bowel syndrome, ulcerative colitis, liver disease, peptic ulcer disease, pancreatitis, viral hepatitis, and hemorrhoids.

In the US, 60 to 70 million people have some type of digestive problem. The most common digestive disorder for women in the US is esophageal reflux, which is felt by 21.1% of the country's female population. Abdominal hernia comes next, followed by irritable bowel syndrome, constipation, and gallstones.

It is imperative for busy women to check on their digestive health and know what their lifestyle and eating habits are causing their digestive system. The first signs of having a problem is having regular heartburn. Bloating or flatulence due to gas is another symptom to look out for. It may sound a bit gross, but you also need to check on your stool to know whether you are up for a digestive problem or not. If you see blood, undigested food, or oil, then you might want to take note and ask for some professional advice. Diarrhea and constipation, as well as stomach pain when eating or defecation, vomiting, and belching are all symptoms of having some kind of digestive problem.

There are many causes for digestive issues, including health problems that contribute to how our digestive system reacts or functions. Food allergies, the body's inability to absorb nutrients properly, lactose intolerance, infections and issues in your immune system, intestinal wall deterioration, and other allergies are risk factors.

If you have digestive issues, juicing is the most wonderful thing that has been invented for you. Because you have problems digesting your food effectively, juicing makes it possible for you to take in essential nutrients without having to worry about indigestion. The digestion is actually done for you before you drink the juice.

For a more effective juicing that will promote good digestion, you must include the pulp to your juice because it contains the needed fiber for your intestines and stomach. Fiber helps cleanse your digestive system and thus prevents problems in the future.

Vegetable juice is best for those who have digestive issues or are conscious of their digestive health since fruit juice contains a lot of fructose. Starchy vegetables also contain higher levels of sugar than green, leafy or non-starchy veggies. But for those who love fruits, a good juicing recipe for digestion is a combination of 4 kiwifruit, ¼ lime, 2 medium sized apples, 1 pineapple, ¼ lemon with rind, and 2 peeled oranges juiced together. This is best served cold as a refreshing juice drink.

For whatever particular purpose you have when juicing, always base your recipes on the basics of your objective (Are you juicing to prevent cancer? What causes cancer, then? What things should you avoid? What type of vitamins and minerals help in preventing cancer?) And how it can be achieved (Where can these powerful vitamins and minerals be found?). Effective juicing can be done through correct knowledge and information, as well as continuous and regular intake of the right vegetable and fruit juices combined with proper meals and diet. By doing so, you can be sure that your body is well-nourished, armed with strong immune system, and functions well to eliminate all the bad elements that you intake in all sorts of activities.

Women should particularly be aware of what juicing can do to their bodies once it is done correctly. So before you begin juicing, make sure you are well-familiar with yourself first—know your body, your lifestyle, your mood and disposition, and your whole personality so that you can practice the right juicing habits. Remember, juicing must not make you feel unsatisfied. Rather, it should make you feel powerful, healthy, and contented. So if you are feeling a bit (or totally) deprived when you start juicing, you may want to start over and begin with the first steps to make sure you are doing it right. Otherwise, it may not do you any good as you expect.

Chapter 8: Food Combining

* * *

Food combining is the act of putting two or more types of food together to create a recipe. It may be good or bad for your health, depending on the particular characteristics of each food that you integrate in your recipe. We have already discussed how we can experiment on our favorite vegetables and fruits when juicing, and have constantly brought up the need to properly exercise juicing with the right diet—that which involves real, solid food. Juicing alone does not often causes unlikely effects such as that which were mentioned in the previous chapters. So keep in mind that unless you are doing it as a temporary and weight-losing program, juicing without eating proper meals will bring you problems instead of solutions.

There is a proper combination of foods that will not make you suffer from indigestion or some other kind of digestion problem. Between vegetables and fruits or both, you must know what to and what not to combine. Between juicing and proper meals, you must be able to combine the right stuff to avoid high cholesterol, malnutrition, clogged arteries, gallstones, and other disorders such as food allergies and diarrhea, bloating, heartburn, weight gain, constipation, leaky gut syndrome, and many more.

The combination of acid and alkali (or starchy foods and protein-rich foods), for example, is a bad food combination that will surely make you feel uncomfortable if not fully unable to function well.

Proper food combining allows for easy and ideal digestion, which in turn keeps you away from undigested food inside your stomach. Indigestion or the inability to digest your food properly will leave toxic waste inside your body, and results in nausea, stomach pain, and bloating. You would not want this to happen as you attend that special event in your best evening gown, so keep an eye on the food that you eat!

The usual American meal made of steak, potatoes, soda, and bread is a suicide when it comes to proper food combining. As you get to your favorite restaurant, you start off with a cold soda which basically holds up your stomach's act of digesting whatever you are about to take. As you eat your bread, your digestive system focuses on it and forgets about your steak and potato as you eat them next. In a standstill, your stomach will then make you feel so full, bloated, and gassy.

Now, don't go believing that combining meat with fiber (fruits and vegetables) is always the right way to food combining. Eating fruits after a meal can also cause gas and bloating, contrary to what we commonly think. People think that eating a fruit or fruits after a heavy meal helps their bodies digest the heavy part. However, the contrary happens because fruits have fructose which is easy to process without the need for digestion. On the other hand, carbohydrates or protein need much more time to get digested and processed, and affects the fruit that you eat after your meal. Instead of being expelled sooner, the fruit will stay in your stomach for a longer period of time and will ferment. This is why you will get gas by doing this wrong habit.

Another bad habit wrongfully done in most cultures is the combination of protein-rich ingredients or food such as with cheese and egg omelets. Combining starchy foods with protein such as in lasagna or sandwiches is another common mistake done in western or European culture. The combination of tomato sauce and cheese in pasta, pizza, or other Mexican dishes is a no-no if you want optimum digestion. Juice, which is acidic, and milk or other forms of dairy are two incompatible ingredients that can diminish your ability to digest, and has the ability to cause allergies, sinusitis, colds, and cough. It is also a known cause of the production of toxins inside the body, so make sure you avoid yogurt with fruits, or oatmeal with milk and juice. Mixing melon fruit with milk is also not a good idea.

Good and Bad Food Combinations

"So what options do I have?" Surely, this is a question that is boggling your mind right now. All the food combinations that you believed were alright since they tasted like heaven are actually creating hell inside your digestive system.

Do not worry, as there are still a lot of choices left even if you start taking out these unhealthy food combinations on your daily recipes. There is still even a lot more options even as you introduce juicing to your body, and combine it with proper meals.

Food combining allows you to get all the important nutrients that you need. If you stick with one particular type of food, you may develop deficiency of other nutrients that are not present in your chosen food. A number of vegetables have most vitamins and minerals in them, but if you are seeking for a particular effect of juicing, not all vegetables may give the most positive results.

Whether you are into juicing fruits or vegetables, there is a good combination that will help you get your ultimate objective. Unlike what most people think, mixing just any type of fruits together does not instantly make a healthy juice drink. You may be thinking that you are on a fruit diet but behind everything, you can be causing damage to your digestive system.

The basic rule when combining fruits is to avoid mixing acid fruits and sweet fruits together. Acid fruits take up to 2 hours to digest. Examples of these fruits are cranberries, grapefruits, sour apples, sour peaches, sour plums, loganberry, pomegranate, tomatoes, lime, current, orange, lemon, tangerine, pineapple, tangelo, and strawberries. Sweet fruits include bananas, mangoes, dates, raisin, fig, all dried fruits, papaya, persimmon, prunes, and sapote.

It is okay to combine acid fruits or sweet fruits with sub-acid fruits like apricots, boysenberries, apples, blackberries, blueberries, cherimoyas, cherries, grapes, elderberries, huckleberries, fresh figs, guavas, kiwis, nectarines, mulberries, peaches, plums, passion fruits, pears, quince, prickly pear, and raspberries.

All kinds of melons (like Casaba, Cantaloupe, Banana melon, Christmas melon, Crenshaw melon, Persian melon, Honeydew melon, Watermelon, Nutmeg melon, and Muskmelon) are best eaten alone. They usually take at most two hours to digest.

Although fruits are commonly added to make our meals taste more enjoyable, they are best eaten on their own. Experts say that if you want to have regular snack, you can eat fruits on an empty stomach since they are easy to digest and doing so will prevent difficulties in digesting food.

Vegetables are classified into two categories: starchy and non-starchy veggies. Low and non-starchy vegetables are okay to combine with protein starch that comes from beans, soy beans, peas, and navy beans. You can also mix non-starchy vegetables with protein fat from dairy products, avocado, nuts and seeds, olives, and butter, cream, and oils. Protein starch and fat take as much as 12 hours to digest, just like meat and poultry. This is why when you eat a whole steak on your date, you will feel somewhat full until the next morning (or maybe until lunch!) since that piece of meat is giving your stomach a hard time doing its job.

Non-starchy vegetables are green, leafy ones, and bamboo shoots, bell pepper, cabbage, cauliflower, broccoli, eggplant, mung bean sprouts, mushrooms, okra, radish, turnip, sea vegetables, artichokes, alfalfa sprouts, beets, Brussels sprouts, asparagus, chard, carrots, leeks, garlic, scallions and many more.

Starchy vegetables take up to five hours before they get digested, just like non-starchy vegetables. They are fine when combined with the latter, since they practically take the same amount of time to digest. Anything that has a lot of carbohydrates, potatoes, squash, chestnuts, pumpkin, corn, grains, and Jerusalem artichoke are examples of starchy vegetables that you should not combine with meat and poultry, as well as protein-rich dairy and even fruits. After all, fruit and vegetable intermixing should be avoided unless you are prepared for some gaseous experience!

Take a look at how you usually eat—what type of food you prepare for breakfast, lunch, dinner, and in-between snacks. You will realize that without knowing it, you have been causing problems for your digestive system.

The typical idea of a "healthy meal" for an American is balancing the go, grow, and glow foods (carbohydrates, protein, and vegetables or fruits). This is seen is such a way that people just try to look for options when preparing their meals, and not scrutinize them effectively. For so long, even during our younger years, health-conscious people who do not get proper education about food combining take so much time and effort in choosing their foods and preparing their meals, but people often eat oatmeal with milk and banana during breakfast, and they think they have fed themselves with a healthy combination of starch, fruits, and dairy. Quite oppositely, milk and banana combinations are considered toxic-producing food combinations and slows down the body and mind's reaction. It is very difficult to digest milk and bananas altogether, so make sure that if you use this combination, choose to very ripe banana and add some nutmeg and/or cardamom to support digestion. Meanwhile, it is better to eat the oatmeal with milk and banana separately to avoid this problem. As fruits are best taken with an empty stomach, you can eat the banana ahead of time, and wait 30 minutes before eating your oatmeal.

If you are to practice juicing with regular meals, the correct combination of your daily juicing recipe and regular meals should be based on the right food combination we have discussed earlier.

If you are pregnant, or planning to get pregnant, juicing can cause you harm if you do not combine it with the right food match, or you are unable to balance your intake of the different types of fruits and vegetables. It is vital to ensure that you get complete nutrition for your health and your baby's. Therefore, your juicing and overall diet should be balanced, well combined, and planned based on pregnancy's necessities. You need additional folate or folic acid, iodine, iron, calcium, zinc, manganese, vitamin D, vitamin C, vitamin A in varying amounts. You must talk to your ob-gyne regarding the needed nutrients that you must consider as you plan for your meals.

Women who are always on the go should also be conscious about the kind of food that they eat. While they should have more carbohydrate or starch intake, it should be clear that eating pure carbs or starchy vegetables is going to be an unbalanced diet.

Eating chicken or fish with rice or any other food rich in carbohydrates is also unbeneficial to your health. Aside from giving you a lot of reasons to gain weight and lose control of your figure, this weight-adding combination is a wrong choice that may leave you feeling bloated. Worse, you can have indigestion and get other digestive issues.

Bacon and eggs for breakfast represents the biggest killer in preserving a healthy diet. Bacon, aside from being a protein starch and protein fat rich food, has plenty of preservatives, and salt. When fried, it accrues more fats through the cooking oil. If you plan to waste your efforts in juicing to lose weight and return to your healthy self, then fried bacon and eggs will serve you the best results.

Pancakes are also commonly served with bananas or other sweet fruits for breakfast. Skip this as well. Both are high in sugar, and take different amounts of time for digestion, which makes them unhealthy for the busy career woman.

Peanut butter and jelly sandwich for your kids is also not a good idea, although a lot of parents prepare this for their children. Egg and toast, turkey sandwich, bagel and cream cheese are just a few more of the bad food pairings that play a huge role in the deterioration of your health. They are also part of the big syndicate that robs your body of the essential nutrients and cause the increase in toxins and thus lead you towards deadly medical conditions such as cancer, diabetes, and the like.

Now, you might be thinking that you have violated proper food combining all your life. Well, that is no longer surprising since most Americans practice such unhealthy lifestyles that circle on fast food chains and steak houses as they do not have enough time to cook and shop ingredients for themselves. Full time moms may have more chances of changing their family's health through implementing good food combinations. Career women and those who focus on their businesses are in great need of a diet reform—a change in their habits that will start with proper education on how and why food combining is done.

Always keep in mind that in practicing good food combination, it is imperative to take away bad and unhealthy habits that will keep you from its potential benefits. Food combining and juicing are just two of the things you can do to help keep your body healthy. They, alone, are not enough to keep you healthy. You cannot expect to live long through proper food matching and regular juicing if you smoke cigarettes or drink excessive alcohol. The thing is, you just can't be healthy and live an unhealthy lifestyle at the same time.

Food combining is a good step towards a brighter and happier future. It enables you to build and maintain your body consciously. On the other hand, bad eating habits contravene the advantages and positive effects of proper food combining. There are a lot of these bad habits, but here are some to name a few:

Overindulging in fatty and starchy foods makes it hard for your body to produce enough juices needed to digest the amount of food you have taken. Limit your intake of fatty food and starchy fruits and vegetables, as well as carbohydrate rich grains and products. Do not take them together.

Drinking more than a small number of sips as you eat your meals interferes with your digestive system's enzyme secretion. It dilutes the enzymes that are responsible for the efficient digestion of your meal.

Stress eating, eating when you are tired, eating even when you are not hungry, and forcing yourself to eat foods that you really do not like also stops your body from benefiting well from food combining and juicing.

Eating before you are ready (or your stomach is ready) is another bad habit that counters your efforts in food combining and/or juicing. You can say that you are not yet ready for another meal if you are familiar with the length of time needed to digest all types of food. If you ate steak during your previous meal, make sure your stomach has completely digested (or at least close to it) the meat before eating another piece of meat. If you ate sweet or acidic fruits right after you ate your steak, you are probably suffering from fermenting debris in your stomach and therefore must not force yourself to eat.

Not chewing your food properly, or simply eating too quickly are both included in the list of bad habits which may interfere with your healthy routine.

Sleeping right after eating, as well as vigorously exercising will keep you away from your objectives as to why you are presently into juicing and food combining. The intake of too much seasonings and toxic irritants like onions, pepper, vinegar, and bitter herbs destroys your stomach's natural pH. Taking medicine is also a factor.

There are many things that food combining can bring and supplement juicing, but it is undeniably true that some dietitians and writers say that there is no need for food combining. Their reason boils down to one thing: they say that the human stomach was designed to digest about anything regardless of combination.

Still, we believe that humans have long spoken about their bodies based on real life experiences. Our bodies are not perfect, and they do not function the same. Depending on our particular health conditions, our stomachs work in different efficiency levels. Some stomachs are more sensitive and cannot tolerate too much protein, while some are able to digest them.

Food combining is a customizable program that you can adjust according to your personal needs without foregoing the basics.

After achieving your short term goal (let's say, lose weight), one of the best next goals in food combining is to attain a good disposition in life. This will prevent you from getting stressed, depressed, and therefore eating against your health.

There are many reasons why an average American woman should learn and practice proper food combining. The top of the list says that there is actually nothing to lose and everything to gain when you carefully monitor your diet. After all, as they commonly say, "you are what you eat". If you carelessly indulge in fatty, protein rich, sweet, and acidic foods, then your current personality shows that you do not care about your health. That being said, it is easy to say that you do not care about other people's health as well.

Our generation and the next generations need to know how to combine their foods correctly. Otherwise, they will go on believing that as long as they eat fruits and vegetables, and a good amount of carbs and protein, they will be fine.

No woman should suffer another day from weight gain, indigestion, inadequate supply of nutrients, and different types of avoidable and preventable illnesses. You can start as early as today and begin choosing the things you buy and eat in order to show how much you really care for your body (and for the environment and the whole human race as well!).

Bear in mind that food combining is an essential key to effective juicing. While it seems to be a whole separate complex idea that should be learned and practiced separately, food combining and juicing go well together and can be used to make each other more fulfilling and bear more concrete results.

Chapter 9. My Juicing Cheat Sheet

* * *

J uicing is the word in health these days. But to beginners, blending their first few glasses can be a daunting task. There are simply so many herbs, fruits, and produce to choose from. All of them are rich in vitamins, minerals and nutrients that cleanse your body and revitalize your life. But which ones do you really need? Which combinations of nature's best produce would benefit you the most?

If you are at a loss for answers, no worries! This chapter is all about mastering your juicing menu with a personal juicing cheat sheet that lists down your choices and what good they do for your body. I have listed everything alphabetically and grouped them into fruits, vegetables (sea vegetables are also included), sprouts, nuts and herbs to make it as simple as possible.

Fruits

Fruits are naturally low in fat, sodium, on calories. They are also excellent sources of potassium, fiber, folic acid, vitamin C and other nutrients designed to make you better and stronger. While others will give words of caution about the sugar content of fruits, let us get one thing straight. Any fruit is better than none. And any fruit is far better than a piece of candy when your sweet tooth begins to crave. But if you are really worried about the sugar content, always strive for a variety of fruits and vegetables to make sure you get a good balance of nutrients.

Name of Fruit	Why it is Good for You?
Apple	Apples are rich in vitamin C, iron, magnesium, phosphorus, magnesium and trace minerals. Juice this fruit for a natural immune boost. You also get a good dose of fiber that is good for the digestive tract.
Apricot	Apricots are low in fat, high in fiber, and rich in vitamins C B5, and E, potassium, and beta-carotene. Not only are apricots yummy, they are good for your eyes, your heart, and digestive tract.
Avocado	Avocados brim with leutein, potassium, protein, vitamin E, iron, and

	good fats. They are delicious and versatile! Plus, avocados are rich in heart healthy monounsaturated fats and omega-three fatty acids. Good for the liver, and naturally lowers cholesterol. As a point of clarification, avocados are used for smoothies rather than juicing. But they do blend well with vegetable juices.
Bananas	Bananas are used for smoothies rather than juicing. Packed with potassium that protects the heart against high blood pressure and stroke. They are also a good source of iron, magnesium, vitamins B5 and B6, and vitamin C. Bananas help the heart, digestion, fat burn, and reduce risks for colorectal and kidney cancer.
Bell peppers	Bell peppers are usually classified as a vegetable, but this fruit is good for your heart, strengthens the immune system, protects against types of cancers, and oddly enough, fights sunburns. They are rich in beta-carotene, folate, vitamins C, B1, B2, B3, B5, B6, E and K, phytochemicals, and antioxidants. Please note that the orange, yellow and red should be used, the green variety is still unripe.
Blackberry	Blackberries contain vitamins C, B5, E, K, beta-carotene, phytonutrients, folate, iron, magnesium, and zinc. Blackberries fight free radicals in the body associated with heart disease and cancer. It also helps speed up fat burn.
Blueberry	Called a super food because it is rich in antioxidants and phytonutrients, blueberries are also rich in vitamins C and K, fiber, manganese, and iron. Since they are loaded with vitamins, blueberries also help prevent illness and certain types of cancer.
Cantaloupe	This fruit is a good source of beta-carotene, folate, potassium, and fiber. It also has high levels of vitamins C and B. Cantaloupes help prevent degenerative diseases that bog down the body, ideal for cleansing, rehydrating, and reducing inflammation.
Cherimoya	A cherimoya tastes like a burst of strawberry, mango, and pineapple. It offers vitamins C, B1, B2, B3, B5, and B6, folate, iron, magnesium, phosphorus, potassium, omega-three fatty acids, and fiber. Cherimoyas are good for the heart and the brain. It also boosts immunity, prevents certain types of cancer, fights against osteoporosis, and Parkinson's disease.
Cherry	Not everybody appreciates the tartness of cherry juice, but there is good reason to. Cherries are packed with nutrients such as vitamin C, magnesium, and iron. Because it is rich in antioxidants and anti-

	inflammatory agents, cherries promote body detoxification and boosts colon and heart health.
Cranberry	Cranberry juice is an excellent source of vitamin C, oxalic acids, and dietary fiber. Those with urinary tract infections, respiratory disorders, kidney stones, heart disease and some types of cancer are prescribed to drink cranberry juice.
Cucumber	Although some confuse cucumbers to be vegetables, they are actually fruit. They contain vitamins A, C, K and B5, calcium, potassium and iron. Cucumbers are good for your skin, hair, and nails. They aid in digestion and help prevent cancer. Plus, it promotes weight loss.
Dates	Nutrient-dense dates contain vitamins B5, B3, B2, beta-carotene, potassium, magnesium, phosphorus, calcium, iron, and fiber. Dates are good for the brain, heart and digestive health. They are also good for pregnancy.
Figs	A good source of vitamins B1, B5, B6, beta-carotene, calcium, manganese, iron, and calcium. Figs are low-calorie fruits that get high ratings from weight watchers. They are also a low-intensity laxative that is good for intestinal cleansing even for children.
Durian	Despite the pungent small, there is good reason to eat durian for its nutritional content. Durian is a good source of vitamins C, B1, B2, B3, B5, B6, folate, manganese, potassium, sulfur, magnesium, phosphorus, and iron. Durian has a warming effect on the body that is great for sleeping. It is also good for bone and digestive health, increased immunity, and cancer protection.
Grapefruit	Grapefruit is rich in vitamins C, E, A, folate, niacin, pantothenic acid, pyridoxine, riboflavin, thiamin, potassium, calcium, iron, magnesium, phosphorus and zinc. Because the grapefruit is rich in nutrients, it makes the body stronger by protecting against heart disease and certain types of cancers. Plus, the fruit aids in weight loss.
Grapes	Grapes contain health-protecting antioxidants, including resveratrol and flavonoids. It also has a chockfull of nutrients such as Vitamins C, E, A, K, sodium, potassium, calcium, iron, magnesium, phosphorus and zinc. Grapes maintain healthy blood pressure and prevent certain cancers.
Jackfruit	Jackfruits contain beta-carotene, vitamins C, B2 and B6. These fruits are good for digestive health and can also be used as a natural laxative.
Jujube	The jujube is rich in vitamin C, potassium, phosphorus, manganese,

	calcium, sodium, zinc, and iron. It boosts the immune system, lowers blood pressure; relieves stress and anxiety. It is also a natural sedative and has been known to cure some liver diseases.
Kiwi	Kiwis have a delicious flavor and do the body good. Kiwis are packed with vitamins C, K, E, folate, iron, and potassium. They are excellent for digestion and skin health, and help remove excess sodium buildup.
Kumquat	Kumquats look like small oval oranges. You eat it whole, including the skin. Kumquats have a high percentage of vitamin C, and a good source of calcium, beta-carotene and magnesium. They boost the immune system and helps fight against types of cancer.
Lemon	A lemon is rich in vitamins C, E, A; folate, niacin, pantothenic acid, pyridoxine, riboflavin and thiamin. It also contains sodium, potassium, calcium, iron, magnesium, phosphorus and zinc. Call it a super food if you will! Lemon juice stimulates the digestive tract, aids digestion, supports weight loss, promotes nerve and heart health, prevents kidney stones, and fights cancer.
Limes	Limes contain vitamin C, niacin, pantothenic acid, riboflavin and thiamin. It is also a good source of potassium, iron, magnesium and phosphorus. Limes help reverse the signs of aging and promote overall health. They are good for detox, as well as digestive, blood, nerve and heart health. Also good for cancer protection.
Longans	Longans are a good source of vitamins A and C; iron, magnesium, phosphorus, and potassium. Longans are good for heart and blood health. They boost energy, and are also known to be good beauty and sex tonic. Always remember to remove the black pit before juicing.
Loquat	A loquat is an excellent source of vitamins C and A, pyridoxine, riboflavin, and thiamin. It is also a good source of sodium, potassium, calcium, iron, magnesium, phosphorus, selenium, and zinc. Enjoy its benefits for digestive, skin, and bone health. It is also good for cancer prevention and aids weight loss.
Lychees	Lychees are delicious, delectable, and good for your body. They contain vitamin C, polyphenols, iron, phosphorus, magnesium and potassium. Studies have shown that lychees prevent the growth of cancer cells. It is also immune boosting and helps in weight loss.
Mamey Sapote	Contains vitamins C, A, E; folate, calcium, iron, copper, magnesium, manganese, potassium, and zinc. It helps in weight loss and cardiovascular health.
Mangoes	Good source of vitamin C, beta-carotene, calcium and potassium.

	This fruit is good for renal, digestive and blood health. Also helps supports immune system.
Mangosteen	Mangosteen is high in fiber, folate, and vitamins A and C. Many claim to have benefited from its antimicrobial and antiviral benefits. It helps protect against allergies, cancer, pain, high blood pressure, and inflammation.
Nectarines	Nectarines are a rich source of beta-carotene, potassium, fiber, vitamins C, B3, and E. It contains antioxidants that help protect against cancer and other diseases by reducing cellular damage within the body.
Olives	Olives are rich in monounsaturated fats, calcium, phosphorus, vitamins D and A. It also contains flavonoids and polyphenols that reduce inflammation in the body. It is good for those suffering from gastritis and ulcers; and helps prevent rickets and osteoarthritis.
Oranges	Orange juice is the go-to drink for those in need of an immune boost. It contains one hundred seventy phytonutrients and more than sixty known falconoid. These two reduce inflammation, shrink tumors, and prevent blood clots. Oranges are also good in preventing cancers, heart problems, strokes, and constipation.
Papaya	Papayas are extremely dense in beta-carotene, vitamin C, potassium, calcium, phosphorus, and iron. Juicing papaya brings many benefits. It is good for the skin, for indigestion, constipation, irregular menstruation, and helps fight cancer.
Peaches	In this fruit is a chockfull of vitamins C and A; lutein, lycopene, potassium, fiber, and niacin. Peaches are tough cancer fighters, it is also an antioxidant that protects against heart disease and macular degeneration.
Pear	Pears have high content of vitamins C and E, as well as fiber, iodine, and copper. These make pears a source of powerful antioxidants that boost immunity and help prevent diseases such as cancer, high cholesterol, high blood pressure, and inflammatory conditions.
Persimmon	Benefit from its content of vitamin C, fiber, potassium, and antioxidants. Persimmons aid in digestion, help overall wellbeing, and promote liver health and body detoxification.
Pineapple	Pineapples are loaded with vitamin C and various nutrients that help the body fight off disease, including cancer. They also contain a powerful enzyme called bromelain that acts as an inflammatory, aiding in the prevention of arthritis, swelling, carpal tunnel, gout, and sinusitis.

Plums	Plums are a good source of fiber, oxalic acid, beta-carotene, antioxidants, phosphorus, potassium, as well as vitamins A, C, K, B6. Juicing plums can help the body with weight loss, iron absorption, smooth bowel movement, and strengthening the immune system.
Pomegranate	Pomegranate juice is an excellent source of antioxidants like polyhpenols, tannins, and anthocyanins. Studies show that it fights prostate cancer and effective in lowering blood pressure. It is also good for the skin, urinary tract, and overall health.
Raspberries	This fruit is high in vitamins C, K, A, and rich in potassium ellagic acid, magnesium, and phosphorus. Because of its high nutrient content, it is known to lower cholesterol, slow down cancer, and prevent cardiovascular problems.
Sapote	A cup of sapote contains essential Vitamin C, calcium, and phosphorus that promote health and wellbeing.
Strawberry	Strawberries are rich in vitamin C, folate, potassium, vitamins, and minerals. They are known to protect against Alzheimer's disease, reduce bad cholesterol, and prevent certain types of cancers. Strawberries also relieves sore muscles and stress.
Tangerine	Tangerines help you hydrate because of its high water content. High amounts of vitamins A and C boost the immune system and help fight infections. They also provide the body with beta-carotene, calcium, magnesium, and potassium.
Tomato	Apart from being rich in vitamins C, K, B1, B5, and B6, tomatoes contain a powerful antioxidant called lycopene, which protects the liver, lungs, prostate gland, skin, and colon. Scientific studies about lycopene show that it helps prevent macular degeneration, lowers cholesterol, and prevents cancer.
Watermelon	Naturally-packed with vitamin C, beta-carotene, riboflavin, niacin, potassium, sodium, zinc, lycopene and a bunch of other nutrients. These help you stay healthy while reducing the risk of ovarian and cervical cancer. It also helps you shed extra pounds.

Vegetables

Vegetables are packed with enzymes, nutrients, vitamins, and minerals crucial to overall health and wellbeing. Juicing is a great way to get these nutrients into your body, and an excellent means of getting your recommended dose of vegetable servings each day.

Name of Vegetable	Why it is Good for You?
Asparagus	Contains vitamins C, B1, B2, and B3, plus beta-carotene, folic acid, and fiber. It is a natural diuretic and laxative, good for the heart, and great for the kidneys.
Beets	Your digestive system and kidneys will thank you for consuming beets. It has copper, magnesium, iron, potassium, and manganese.
Bok Choy	Rich in antioxidants, vitamins A and C, beta-carotene, calcium, and fiber.
Broccoli	Known as a super food! It is nutrient-dense and protects against types of cancer, promotes healthy vision, and helps body detox.
Cabbage	Its high fiber content aids in digestion. It also has yttrium and selenium that cleanses the mucous membrane of the stomach and intestinal tract.
Carrot	Carrots are excellent sources of beta-carotene, potassium, and selenium. They help eye function, infections, improve liver function, and help protect against cancer.
Cauliflower	They are nutrient-dense and full of antioxidants. As a tip though, juice the base and not the florets.
Celery	Celery is high in organic sodium, magnesium, and iron that help cleanse the digestive system of uric acid. It also has vitamin C that helps in cancer prevention.
Chard	Has a healthy amount of vitamins C, K, E, beta-carotene, copper, iron, magnesium, manganese, phosphorus, potassium, selenium, sodium, and zinc.
Chlorella	Though it is an algae, it is considered a super food. It is anti-cancer and good for detoxification.
Collards	Collards are rich in chlorophyll, antioxidants, and other nutrients. It also has good amounts of vitamins C, K, B1, B2, B3, B5, and B6. Collard greens protect against hemorrhoids and colon cancer.
Corn	Yes, corn can be juiced. Just be careful to choose organic corn and avoid genetically modified ones. Corn has vitamins C, B1, B2, B3, B5, and B6, as well as other good-for-you nutrients. Not too much though as it is high in sugar.
Dandelion	The bitter dandelion greens are excellent blood cleansers, detoxifiers, and digestive aid. They are a source of vitamins C, B1, B2, B6, K and E, beta-carotene, folate, calcium, fiber, sodium, and omega six.
Dulse	It is a nutritional powerhouse of vitamins, beta-carotene, iodine, potassium, and zinc. A quarter ounce of dulse contains thirty percent

	of your daily dose of iron. A cup of dulse can give you up to six grams of protein.
Jicama	A jicama is sweet to the taste and high in fiber that has zero calories. Ideal for weight watchers and diabetics.
Kale	Some also call kale a super food as it is an excellent source of chlorophyll, calcium, iron, sulfur, beta-carotene, and a chockfull of vitamins. It fights inflammation, prevents cancer, and helps the body detox.
Kelp	Kelp is high in minerals, folate, iron, calcium, zinc, sodium, phosphorus, copper, and vitamins K and E.
Lettuce	Dark green varieties of lettuce (and not iceberg lettuce) are a good source of chlorophyll. It is mostly water and contains vitamins, folate, potassium, iron, calcium and other nutrients.
Nori	You should add nori or laver to your juicing list as it is nutrient and vitamin dense. It boosts immunity with high content of beta-carotene and vitamins C, B1, B2, B3, B5, B6, and E.
Okra	Okra soothes the digestive tract by coating the intestines and acting as a natural lubricant. It is good for people with digestion problems, but do not use more than one okra per quart or it can change the consistency of your juice.
Onions	Onions are natural detoxifiers, antiseptics, and stimulants. Add a little bit of onion into your juice from time to time to reap the rewards of its nutrient-dense contents.
Parsnip	Parsnips are a great source of folate, fiber, manganese, copper, and vitamins C, E, B1, and B5. They are known to detox and cleanse the body.
Peas	Peas can go into your juice too! They add protein, vitamins, minerals, and nutrients into your concoction.
Peppers	Peppers can boost the metabolism, making it a great fat-burner. They also contain beta-carotene, vitamins C and B6, copper, iron, manganese, magnesium, and omega six.
Pumpkin	Pumpkins reduce inflammation. They also lower risks for lung and prostate cancer. Plus, they are a good source of beta-carotene, vitamins B2, C, and E, copper, iron, and potassium.
Radish	Those with thyroid, liver, and stomach problems will benefit from radish. They also aid in weight loss by adding to the feeling of fullness. Radish has a generous amount of folate, vitamin C, copper, iron, and zinc.
Spinach	Spinach is very dense in nutrients. It is good for the blood because of

	its iron and chlorophyll content. It is also rich in vitamins B2 and B6, minerals, iron, and potassium.
Spirulina	This is another algae that is considered a super food. It is chlorophyll-rich, digestible, antibacterial, anti-fungal, and immune boosting.
Squash	Winter squash is great for the eyes and heart. It is a cancer-fighter because of its high beta-carotene content. It is also dense in vitamins B1, B5, B6, and C, copper, iron, magnesium, manganese, phosphorus, and potassium.
Sweet potato	Sweet potatoes are natural detoxifiers, support digestion, anti-cancer, and good for the body. They contain beta-carotene, vitamins B1, B5, B6, copper, iron, magnesium, manganese, phosphorus, and potassium.
Turnip	Turnips help fight cancer and are known for anti-biotic and anti-viral benefits. The bottom line is that they make your body stronger.
Wakame	An excellent source of beta-carotene, vitamins E, B1, B2, B3, B5folate, and omega three.
Zucchini	Good to eat, good to juice. Has vitamins C, B, A; lutein, folate, and potassium.

Sprouts

You should consider adding sprouts to your juice. Sprouts are easily digested and concentrated with enzymes, proteins, vitamins, and minerals. Get used to their flavor by adding small amounts to your juice before adding them by the handful.

Name of Sprout	Why it is Good for You?
Adzuki	Adzuki sprouts are highly nutritious and rich in vitamins B1 and C; protein, niacin, iron, magnesium, zinc, calcium.
Alfalfa	Alfafa is loaded with beta-carotene and vitamins B1, B2, B3, B5, B6, C, D, E, K. It helps against blood clotting and helps the body fight disease.
Barley grass	Barley is said to be the only vegetable on Earth that can supply all the nutrients the body needs from birth to old age! It has four times the calcium of milk, twenty-two times the iron in spinach, and as much protein per ounce as a big juicy steak. It helps with longevity, weight loss, an improved immune system, and overall wellbeing.
Buckwheat	Unhulled buckwheat contains a list of vitamins, minerals, and nutrients. It is an antioxidant, anti-inflammatory, diuretic, and a

	fighter of disease.
Chick Pea	Add a bit of chick pea or garbanzo beans for its nutritional content. It contains vitamins B1, B2, B3, B5, B6, K, folate, copper, iron, magnesium, manganese, phosphorus, potassium, zinc, selenium, and omega six.
Fenugreek	Good for the heart and lowers the risk of heart attacks. It is also good for the digestive system and pancreas, balances blood sugar, and dense in beta-carotene.
Green pea	Green peas protect our eyes due to its high beta-carotene content. It is also rich in antioxidants.
Lentil	Lentils are high in protein, minerals, and B vitamins. It is also a good source of fiber that can lower cholesterol.
Mung beans	Mung beans help lower cholesterol, fight against breast cancer by inhibiting growth of cancer cells, diabetic-friendly, and a great source of protein.
Sunflower	Also called a super food, sunflower sprouts are rich in B vitamins, minerals, and good fats; loaded with protein and help build immunity.
Wheat	Add this to your glass for an extra punch of protein, minerals, and vitamins C, E, B1, B2, B3, B5, and B6, minerals.
Wheatgrass	Wheatgrass has extremely high levels of chlorophyll & phytonutrients. It is called a super food because it is a cleanser, purifier, detoxifier, anti bacterial, blood builder, and liver cleanser all in one. It is also rich in beta-carotene, vitamin C, and B complex vitamins.

Nuts

Milk from nuts has become a popular substitute for health enthusiasts. It is lactose-free and packed with nutrients. While making milk from nuts will not really go with your juice, you can use them as a base for smoothies. You can also add some nuts on top of your juice for texture and flavor.

Name of Nut	Health Benefits
Almonds	Almond milk is high in protein, potassium, magnesium, phosphorus, and calcium.
Chestnut	Chestnut milk is low in fat, contains complete B vitamins, and an excellent source of fiber.
Cashew	Cashew milk is high in protein, vitamin A, potassium, and

	magnesium.
Coconut	Coconut milk is a great source of electrolytes, copper, iron, magnesium, manganese, phosphorus, potassium, zinc, iodine, and selenium.
Hazel	Hazelnut milk is delicious and high in protein, calcium, potassium, and sulfur.
Pecans	Pecan milk is good for the heart, with ample amounts of protein, potassium, and vitamin A.
Pine	Enjoy pine nut milk for a good dose of protein, iron, niacin, thiamine, and phosphorus.
Walnuts	Walnut milk is also rich in protein, magnesium, vitamin A, and magnesium.

Herbs

Name of Herb	Health Benefits
Basil	Basil contains vitamins C, A, and B complex, as well as beta-carotene, lutein, and zea-xanthin. It is a known antioxidant, digestive aid, and disease fighter.
Chives	You can use the stems and leaves of chives to take advantage of its nutrient-dense content.
Cilantro	Rich in antioxidants, vitamins, and minerals that keep the body healthy. It also helps flush mercury from the body.
Fennel	Known as a healing herb, fennel helps protect the eye, aids the brain in releasing endorphins, and even suppresses appetite.
Garlic	Because it increases the hormone leptin, garlic is said to control appetite. It is also antifungal, antiviral, anti-parasitic, and antibacterial.
Ginger Root	Adding ginger to your juice helps boost metabolism and strengthens the immune system.
Mint	Mint adds flavor, and gives a calm and relaxing effect. It is dense with vitamins and minerals, and is said to help relieve headaches.
Nettles	Those with muscle pain, joint pain, and arthritis will benefit from juicing nettles. It is also effective against digestive problems and hemorrhoids.
Oregano	Oregano leaves are antimicrobial and antiviral. It is rich in beta carotene, folate, and vitamins C, B1, B2, B3, B5, B6, E, and K.
Parsley	Rich in beta-carotene, vitamin K, vitamin c, potassium, iron, calcium,

	zinc, sodium, fiber, selenium, manganese, phosphorus, and copper.
Rosemary	Rosemary boosts the immune system, improve circulation, and helps digestion. It is an antiseptic and antimicrobial. And because of its anti-inflammatory properties, it can help against asthma attack.
Thyme	Add thyme if you are dealing with respiratory tract problems. It is antiseptic, antibacterial, and an antioxidant. It also has beta-carotene, folate, iron, and vitamins B2, B3, B5, B6, and C.
Watercress	Highly nutritious, watercress offers many benefits. It is a diuretic, blood purifier, antibiotic, and resistance-booster.

Chapter 10. Discovering Detox Juicing

* * *

Believe it or not, the idea of detox juice cleansing has been around for years—more than a century to be exact. It was in the 1900's that people thought that detoxification would do the body good. They reasoned out that the body was already absorbing toxins from the environment that could lead to disease. But the concept was abandoned in the 1930's when there was no concrete evidence to support juicing claims. Fast-forward more than one hundred years later and the world is flooded with a sea of testimonials about the benefits of juicing. More and more are reaping the rewards of detox juicing, enjoying increased energy and improved health.

Detox juicing benefits the body by eliminating toxins that weaken the immune system and make us prone to degenerative diseases. This chapter aims to answer the why's and how's of detox juicing, and tips on how to kick-start your own detox.

What Toxins Are You Talking About?

We live in a society consumed by fast food, processed foods, and artificially flavored drinks. It seems as though the grit and grind of hectic everyday life has caught up to our bodies. In giving our bodies nutrition from the fastest and easiest sources possible, we have made difficult-to-pronounce chemicals a staple of our everyday diet. These toxins hamper our body's natural ability to balance sugar and metabolize cholesterol. And as we continue to consume them, we turn our bodies into a breeding ground of fat and disease.

A 2009 report by the Centers for Disease Control and Prevention (CDC) on human exposure to environmental chemicals revealed that every person the CDC tested had a host of chemicals inside their body. Shocking, right? This list of toxic cocktails included chemicals from flame-retardants and a hormone-like substance called Bisphenol A (2) found in plastic. Even more shocking was the finding that the average newborn has almost three hundred chemicals found in the umbilical cord.

Below are some of the more common toxins, preservatives, and additives we consume everyday:

Pesticides

Have you heard of the dirty dozen? Apples, celery, peaches, sweet bell peppers, nectarines, strawberries, cherries, pears, grapes, spinach, lettuce, and potatoes are known to have high amounts of pesticides. Choosing organic alternatives to these twelve can reduce your exposure to pesticides by eighty percent.

Pesticides accumulate in our bodies over time. Our bodies cannot remove them even if they do damage to our endocrine, reproductive, circulatory, immune, and central nervous systems. A recent study showed that all of us have dangerous traces of polychlorinated biphenyls (PCBs), dioxin, chlordane, aldrin, dieldrin, and dioxin in our blood streams. Scary!

Sodium nitrate and nitrite

If you love processed foods and meat products, then you expose yourself regularly to sodium nitrate and nitrite. Yes, hotdogs, ham, corned beef, luncheon meat, and many others belong to this list.

Caffeine

Natural caffeine in moderation is fine. But too much (especially if it comes from gum, soda, diet soda, and the link) is addictive, affects fertility, and is even known to cause birth defects, heart conditions, behavioral changes, osteoporosis, and insomnia.

BHA/BHT

If you have the habit of reusing or reheating oil to save a few bucks—stop! Oil that is used again has BHA/BHT that increases appetite, affects sleep, and causes problems to the liver, kidney, heart, and even cancer. Throw old oil away!

Refined Sugar

Never has the world consumed so much candy through sweets, candies, chocolates, cakes—name it! However, this toxic love affair leads to diabetes, weight gain, arthritis, migraines, decreased immunity, gallstones, breast cancer, and heart disease. In fact, many diseases can be linked to too much sugar.

Sugar Sweetened Drinks

Artificial sweeteners like saccharin, aspartame, and NutraSweet affect brain neurochemistry. These are found in soft drinks, sport drinks, and other sweetened beverages.

Monosodium Glutamate or MSG

MSG is not just found in food, even candy, gums, and yoghurt has trace amounts of it. MSG is harmful because it causes obesity and inhibits our natural growth hormone. It also causes headaches, nausea, weakness, and changes in heart rate.

Brominated Vegetable Oil (BVO) and Partially Hydrogenated Vegetable Oil

These two reduce immunity, increase allergic reactions, elevate cholesterol levels, and has even been tied to certain types of cancer. BVO is toxic to children, while Partially Hydrogenated Vegetable Oil is full of trans fat—making it toxic to adults.

Now that you have an idea of the toxins consumed everyday, does it not seem like the world is caught up in a vicious toxic cycle? If you are ready to cleanse and give your body a fighting chance against an unhealthy lifestyle, then get your juicer ready and reap the benefits of detox juicing.

Benefits Of Detox Juicing

The human body is so amazing that it has the ability to cleanse itself of most toxins we consume. We can thank the liver and the kidneys for that. However, with the amount of toxins we are ingesting, detox juicing can step in to combat the effects of an unhealthy way of eating and living. Here are three of its top benefits:

1. Detox juicing means subsisting on pressed juices from fruits and vegetables for a few days. As we know, fruits and vegetables are nutrient-dense! It is an excellent way to get more phytonutrients from vegetables and fruits into your body. Juicing allows you to absorb the nutrients with less digestive work required.

2. It can help you jumpstart a healthy new routine.
3. It eliminates fats, sugar, and processed foods from the diet. Indeed, detox juicing can result in increased energy, clearer skin, and less digestive issues.

As a general and wisdom-filled rule, it is always best to consult your physician before entering any new regimen. And be sure to check that your juicing program gives you all the nutrients calories you need per day.

Getting Started

Juicing provides us with a simple yet satisfying way to end unhealthy eating and reset our metabolism. But before you begin, there are eleven important points to take into consideration.

First, know why you want to do detox juicing.

Your primary motivation must be your own physical wellbeing and flushing out toxins from your system. Do not do it because your friends said so, or because your favorite celebrity endorsed it.

Also, it is no secret that everyone wants to lose extra pounds. But do not make weight loss the moving force behind your juice detox. Fruits can be high in sugar, so you may feel disappointed if you do not get the weight loss results you hoped for. Weight loss follows naturally after you become committed to living and eating clean.

Choose a juice detox program that is right for you.

The standard detox regimen will take two to four days, but a longer detox will have the most beneficial outcome. As mentioned earlier, choose a program that will provide enough nutrients and calories for you to exist without headaches and low morale. In other words, choose a program you know you can stick to! There is nothing worse than binging on a toxic buffet because your four-day juice detox has left you too hungry.

Prepare yourself physically and mentally.

Detoxification is an important and necessary step prior to any program. It is the time to wean yourself from unhealthy habits. For many years, toxins, preservatives, chemicals, and caffeine have found a happy home in our system causing addiction. Think of them like narcotics and nicotine—they are hard to let go of, and if you do find the strength to break free, you should prepare for withdrawal systems.

Give yourself three to five days to prepare for your upcoming detox. This is the usual time people can adjust to changes into their lifestyle and diet. Start by making a list of habits that are causing harm to your body and gradually limit your indulgence of them. A word of caution though—some people get terrible migraines, cramps, or even fall into depression from keeping away the things that they think make their day complete. It could be cigarettes, too much coffee, chips, or chocolate!

Start taking in a lot of fresh fruits and vegetables to ease yourself into the pre-detox process. For example, instead of taking coffee, eggs, and bacon for breakfast, a fresh glass of grapefruit or orange juice and an apple in the morning is a great start. Limit also the amount of fat intake by eating salads with lemon juice and herbs with daily meals cutting down on the amount of fatty or processed foods. Even eating half of your normal daily intake can do wonders.

Plan out your detox.

The first two days on a juice detox will be the hardest. Your body will adjust—and it might even rebel a bit. That is why it is better to start on a Thursday or Friday and continue over the weekend when your workload is low.

Get your goods ready.

Freshness is important when doing detox juicing. Unlike cooking that eliminates a lot of important vitamins and minerals naturally found in fresh fruits and vegetables, juicing lets you take nutrients in quickly and effectively.

One day before your detox, head to the farmer's market or the grocery to buy your fruits and vegetables. Buy the freshest ingredients and avoid canned produce. If you have the time, it is always advisable to buy your fruit and vegetables a day prior to use so you can get the optimum nutrient content. Buying organically grown produce will also ensure that you do not ingest any of the pesticides you are trying to rid your body of. Once you get them home and you are not sure they are organic, do a quick rinse of water with a small amount of vinegar or lemon juice to do the trick.

Detox juicing is a simple and easy way to detoxifying or cleansing yourself. There is no need for elaborate preparations, you simply choose which of nature's gifts to drink today and pop them into your juicer. Preparation time is fast because all you need is a good juicer and a good knife (to cut the large pieces of fruit or vegetables), and you are ready to go. Cut, juice, and drink.

Drink the right amount of juice.

When doing a juicing cleanse, it is recommended that you drink anywhere from thirty-two to ninety-six fluid ounces of juice per day to get the optimal cleansing effect. And drink lukewarm water in between juice intake to help with absorption and toxin elimination. Remember, water is your friend, especially during your juice detox.

Here is an example of how a basic detox juicing regiment might go:

- When you wake up in the morning, drink lukewarm water infused with lemon and cucumbers. This can be prepared the night before.
- A glass of cashew or almond milk.
- Take between eight to twenty-four ounces of juice, four times within the day that includes three servings of green vegetable juice – mix of spinach, kale, celery stalks, romaine lettuce, cucumber with some apple and lemon to taste. Also include one serving of beets, carrot and apple juice within the day.
- End with a glass of cashew or almond milk.

You will start to feel the effects two to three days after you start. And you will feel a whole lot better once the cleansing is done.

The days after your juice cleanse are just as crucial. You should begin slowly re-introducing different foods to your diet. Do this slowly and listen to your body after each intake of food. If a certain food makes you feel sick, it means your body is reacting to. Since cleansing has eliminated the toxins, your body will let you know loud and clear if something does not agree with you.

Stay hydrated.

It is common knowledge that we should drink a lot of water daily. It has so many benefits that you should drink six to eight glasses per day regardless if you are cleansing or not. Water energizes muscles, maintains fluid balance in the bodies, helps our kidneys, and essential for overall health. Plus, it has no preservatives or additives. It is one hundred percent good for the body.

Water is vital to the cleansing process. Drinking a lot of water will help speed up detoxification and will help your body burn fat. It also helps give the feeling of fullness should you get hunger pangs.

Get enough sleep.

When changing one's lifestyle, it is important to get at least eight hours of sleep daily. Some may get by with six hours of rest, but eight will get you the best results. Without proper rest, one may become stressed and mentally exhausted. Stress is a major hindrance during the detoxification process. A lack of sleep can lead to headaches, nausea, and decrease in energy. And while you are set on getting enough hours of sleep, be sure to turn in early as well. Studies show that sleeping before eleven in the evening is optimal for the body to rejuvenate and heal itself.

Are you finding it hard to sleep? Try breathing exercises and meditation to relax your body and wind down.

Conserve energy.

The first few days of a juice detox will be met by challenges. You might feel a bit weak as your body adjusts to your juice intake. That is why most are advised to limit their exercise and training program during the detox regimen. It will only be for a few days anyway, and the benefits of the juice cleanse far outweigh the burden of skipping the gym for two to four days.

Too much strenuous activity can have an adverse effect on you. Your body is scrambling for energy during your detox phase, so if you push it by keeping the intensity level high during your workout you may only be doing yourself more harm than good.

There are acceptable forms of exercise during the detox period: a brisk walk or a light swim is perfectly fine. You can use this alone time to relax and meditate. Massages and other relaxing activities are also encouraged during your cleanse. Remember that being relaxed and rested will boost your body's detox process.

Have a support group.

One of the best ways to succeed in a juice cleanse is to surround yourself with positive and supportive people. A detox buddy or a support group is highly recommended. It could be a family member or a friend who could be doing the same detox program as you are.

Accountability is a big word! It means that you own up to your actions and that you are taking responsibility for your decisions! Having a support group helps you strengthen your resolve to be accountable to your body. Your buddy is there to give you a needed push when you hit a wall and you feel like giving up.

If there is no one you know who could be a support buddy at this time, why not go online and join a health forum? You would be surprised to find how many people are going through the same experience as you are facing now.

Juice on-the-go.

If you are a person who is always on the go, you can still do a detox juicing. It will just take extra preparation and making your juice in advanced. Invest in a few BPA-free containers and prepare all your ingredients the night before. Juice your produce in the morning. Ideally, you should consume your juice within one hour from the time you made them. But you can also bring around a cooler with a lot of ice to keep your juice chilled and fresh. Some have even bought portable juicers and made their health tonics right in the office pantry. Yes, it can be done!

Detox juicing is about giving back to your self. Ultimately, you decide to go on a juice cleanse because you want to do your body good. And with all the benefits of detox juicing, this method is a great way to take back your health and jumpstart a clean and nutrient-rich lifestyle!

Chapter 11. What's For Dessert?

* * *

Ah, the myth of the sweet tooth! Everyone claims to have it at one point or another, and once you do, there is a deep urge to satisfy it! A simple definition of a sweet tooth is a liking, craving, or desire for something with sugar. Over the years, the sweet tooth has been a phrase associated with gluttony for high-calorie sweets that pack fat into your body. But in this chapter, we give a new and healthier meaning to the sweet tooth. You will learn that it is indeed possible to satisfy your sweet tooth without blowing your diet.

Decoding the Myth of the Sweet Tooth

It is natural for humans to like or crave something sweet. Our primal ancestors had a sweet tooth too. But at that time, they satisfied their need for something sweet with a piece of ripe fruit. As society evolved, the discovery of sugar has led to the evolution of the sweet tooth as well. Sweets now come from carbohydrate sources apart from fruits—there are just so many sources of sugar to choose from. Candy, sweets, chocolate, cake, soda—name it!

The sweet tooth has absolutely nothing to do with your teeth. Science tells us that taste perception begins on the tongue and the soft palate. This is the place where our taste buds interact with the food and drinks we ingest. And unfortunately (or fortunately as we will see later on), the tongue is not able to distinguish between simple sugars and chemically based sugar substitutes. Our palate will say that something is sweet regardless if it came from natural sources or otherwise!

But it is not only your tongue that is craving. Studies show that the brain has a large role in our sweet cravings. A laboratory test had rats subsist on a diet that was high in sugar. When the scientists abruptly stopped giving sugar, the rats had withdrawal symptoms. It almost seems like they became addicted to the sugar.

Sugar stimulates the brain to release dopamine, a feel-good brain chemical. This natural-high is what is said to make sweets and sugar so appealing. So when you say you have a sweet tooth, it means that your brain has gotten used to increased dopamine levels. And that is when your sweet tooth comes to play.

There are times, however, when you just want something for the flavor of it. Some sweet cravings can also be traced to lifestyle and upbringing. A certain type of food might remind you of fun childhood memories and it might bring a sense of comfort during difficult times. If this is the case, chances are high that you will give into this craving.

What does giving into your craving mean? Highly processed sugar is an empty calorie with no nutritional content what so ever. Ingesting refined sugar is the leading cause of obesity and diabetes around the world. The rise in the rate of obesity and diabetes in children is alarming. This epidemic has also resulted to a rise in incidents of heart disease, hypertension, and other chronic diseases.

Sadly, it has become almost second nature for us to feed ourselves and our children sugary cereals, snacks, and drinks. So much so that they have become a habit. Fast food is also an unfortunate staple this world has become accustomed too. And that said, a lot of people think that kicking the sweet tooth might be harder than we thought.

The Problem With Sugar

How can something that tastes so good be bad for you? We just read that sugar gives us an energy boost and puts us in a positive mood. The problem is that after the natural high, sugar sends our bodies down to crash and reach for more sugar! You can see where this is headed, and you now have a picture of why many are overweight.

But the bad news about sugar does not stop there.

Sugar is one of the primary sources of calories, specifically fructose corn syrup. You can find it everywhere—soda, processed foods, fruit juices, instant coffee, bottled drinks, pasta sauce, cheese, bread, and just about majority of items at the grocery. The sugar industry is on the rise, and so is obesity.

Glucose is the form of energy that was made from humans. Our body can metabolize glucose without putting burden on the liver. But fructose is metabolized differently. The weight of the work is passed onto the liver, and then what is left over is converted into fat. Too much fructose is the primary cause of non-alcoholic fatty liver, abdominal obesity, and most chronic diseases. And the list does not stop there. Sugar has also been announced the culprit of many other disease such as cancer, cholesterol, diabetes, food allergies, eczema in children, cardiovascular disease, attention deficit disorders, bacterial infection, and osteoporosis.

What is the solution to the problem of sugar? If you cannot shake sugar out from your routine, follow doctors' orders and consume no more than twenty-five grams of fructose per day.

Some people try to quit cold turkey. They just stay away from sugar and hold out as long as they can. But the problem with this is that cravings are the result of imbalances in brain chemistry. You might not be hungry at all, but your mind will crave for something sweet. And that is why no matter how hard you try you seem to find your way back to sugar.

But if you are ready to take your life and health back, you can work to you can do away with sugar without giving up the wonderful taste of sweetness. Avoiding sweetness is not necessary and not natural. You can satisfy your craving without compromising your health!

There are natural sources of sugar we can indulge in, just like our ancestors enjoyed. And all without the ill-side effects of too much processed sugar.

Getting Your Sugar-High From Juicing

Fruits and vegetables are excellent sources of vitamins, minerals, nutrients, and fiber. They also contain naturally occurring sugar that keeps your blood sugar levels in check, and satisfies your brain's craving for dopamine.

When juicing fruits and vegetables, be careful not to use those that have too much sugar content. Identify high-sugar fruits and use a small amount as a natural sweetener. And you can get a lot of flavor by combining different produce. Feel free to use exciting combinations like oranges, mangoes, apples, and grapes. You can also combine strawberries, raspberries, blueberries, and blackberries for a refreshing four seasons berry mix. Adding cucumber to a citrus blend of oranges, lemons, grapefruit, and lime makes for a great cooler. The possibilities are limitless!

And if you do get tired with juicing, you can also rely on freezing fruits and making a delicious sorbet. You can add ice, extra fruit, or nut milk to add flavor and character to your dessert. It all comes out as a healthy, natural, and flavorful dessert!

Here is a list of the most common fruits and vegetables used in juicing with their total sugar contents (based on USDA Nutritional Facts):

Fruits	Total Sugar in grams/ 100 grams
Grapes	15.48
Mango	14.8
Cherries, sweet	12.82
Apples	10.39
Pineapple	9.26
Purple Passion Fruit or Granadilla	11.2
Kiwi fruit	8.99
Pear	9.8
Pomegranate	16.57
Raspberries	4.42
Apricots	9.24
Orange	9.35
Watermelon	6.2
Cantaloupe	7.86
Peach	8.39
Nectarine	7.89
Honeydew melon	14.37
Blackberries	4.88
Sour Cherries	8.49
Tangerine	10.58
Plum	9.92
Blueberries	9.96
Figs	16.26
Grapefruit	6.98
Guava	8.92
Papaya	5.9
Strawberries	4.66
Tomato	2.63
Lemon	2.5
Lime	1.69

Vegetables	Total Sugars in grams/ 100 grams
Beets	6.76

Carrots	4.54
Celery	1.83
Broccoli	1.7
Cucumber	1.67
Swiss Chard	1.1
Lettuce	1.76
Kale or Chard	0
Spinach	0.42

Healthy Alternatives to Sugar

If you really cannot kick the sugar habit, the good news is that there are two natural and organic sugar alternatives that are just as sweet and easy to bake and cook with. Meet xylitol and stevia. While they sound like a chemical substance, they are actually nature's best and sweetest.

You can add these to smoothies and fresh juice if you wish. And if you really want to splurge a bit, you can bake healthy with stevia or xylitol.

Stevia (stevia rebaudiana) is an herb that has been used as a sweetener. Though it tastes bitter in huge amounts, it is actually three hundred times sweeter than sugar! So just a little bit comes a long way, and it is calorie-free and one hundred percent natural. It is an ideal sugar replacement!

Since stevia is three hundred times sweeter than traditional sugar, refer to the conversion chart below before using it to replace sugar:

• One-teaspoon stevia (powered) equals one-cup sugar
• One half-teaspoon stevia equals one-tablespoon sugar
• A pinch of stevia equals one-teaspoon sugar
• One-teaspoon stevia (liquid) equals one-cup sugar
• Six drops liquid stevia equals one-tablespoon sugar
• Two drops liquid stevia equals one-teaspoon sugar

Xylitol, meanwhile, is naturally found in fibrous fruits and vegetables, corn cobs and hardwood trees. Despite the fact it seems difficult to pronounce, it is one of the most natural supplements you can give your body. Our body produces up to fifteen grams of xylitol during normal metabolism. It is also known to be anti-microbial because it is a five-carbon sugar. It also boosts immunity!

Not many know that xylitol is used for oral hygiene products. This is because of its anti-microbial property that inhibits bacteria growth. It also has no after taste and ill-effect.

Both stevia and xylitol are globally approved for human consumption. Take advantage of them! Remove processed sugar from your cooking, baking, and sweetening activities and do your body and health a favor.

Natural Sources of Sugar

This chapter also aims to inform you about natural sweeteners that are close to their whole form. You can also use them for cooking, baking, and making smoothies and juices. These naturally occurring sweeteners are also sweeter than actual processed sugar! It makes you wonder why we never made these healthy alternatives our primary sweeteners in the first place.

Honey

Nature gave us honey for natural sweetness and goodness! It is delicious and fulfills any craving for sugary flavors. Plus, it has a power-packed dose of antioxidant that fights off chronic diseases. Honey is sweeter than sugar, so be scarce in using it.

Agave Nectar

Agave is made from the agave plant. The flavor has a hint of caramel and is a great sweetener. It is also very good for your gut because it contains prebiotics that nourishes intestinal bacteria. Be careful though because it has a high calorie count of sixty calories per tablespoon. But do not worry. You do not need as much, because it is way sweeter than sugar.

Blackstrap Molasses

Molasses are the by-product of sugarcane processing. It is very good for the body because just one tablespoon provides iron, vitamin B6, magnesium, calcium, and antioxidants.

Yacon

A yacon is a plant with edible tubers and leaves. A yacon is sweet and healthy at the same time. It is good for blood-sugar disorders and digestive problems, it stimulates colon health, and helps the body absorbs B vitamins and nutrients. It also has generous amounts of potassium and antioxidants.

Coconut Palm Sugar

Coconut palm sugar or coconut nectar sugar or coconut sugar is naturally sweet and nutrient-dense. As the name suggests, it comes from the coconut blossoms and high in vitamins and minerals.

When You Really Need Chocolate

Chocolate for many is like Achilles' heel—it is our weakness! This is the ultimate go-to destination of the sweet tooth. On cold nights, a cup of hot chocolate would really hit the spot. There are also times that you feel like nibbling on a piece of good chocolate. And once you have some, the brain produces dopamine and you are sent on a sugar high. That is a feel-good moment right there.

Chocolate, especially the dark kind, is good for the health. But too much of it is very potent in making a person fat. Let us face it, chocolate has a lot of sugar.

If you are trying to revamp your lifestyle and eat (or drink) clean, then you can find comfort in a healthier alternative to chocolate. Yes there is, and it is called cocoa nibs.

Cocoa nibs are cocoa beans that have been roasted, separated from the husk, and broken down into smaller pieces. You can eat them as a snack, add them to your baking ingredients, or top them on smoothies.

As you will soon see, there are many reasons why you should eat them for your next chocolate craving! Cocoa nibs are flavorful, nutritious, and brimming with benefits. Here are a few of them:

- Just one ounce of it contains one hundred thirty calories, thirteen grams of fat, three grams of protein, and ten grams of carbohydrates.
- It is also an excellent source of potassium, magnesium, calcium, iron, copper, and zinc. Not to mention it is high in antioxidants that protect the body from diseases.

- Cocoa nibs contain theobromine, a central nervous system stimulant that is a bit like caffeine. Nonetheless, it can give you a much-needed energy boost during the day.
- Cocoa nibs can make you feel happier! It contains tryptophan that produces serotonin. Increased serotonin levels help improve mood and relieve anxiety.
- It can release endorphins into your system! Those are happy hormones right there.
- Cocoa nibs can help relieve premenstrual syndrome or PMS due to its magnesium content. Magnesium deficiency is common before a woman's monthly period. It is what sends women to seek chocolate while they experience PMS.
- It contains good fats! The healthy monounsaturated fats found in cocoa nibs help improve levels of good cholesterol.
- Cocoa is a natural source of flavanols, antioxidants that improve blood circulation, reducing risks of blood clots, strokes, and heart attacks.
- Because cocoa nibs contain chromium, it helps stabilize blood sugar levels and control appetite.

A word of advice: Cacao is best eaten raw. Your digestive system can maximize its vitamins, minerals, and antioxidants in its raw form.

Tips to Fending Off Your Sweet Tooth

Earlier, we discussed how sugar levels and an imbalance in brain chemistry trigger sugar cravings. So you are perfectly normal, and you can take comfort knowing that many others experience the same sweet cravings as you.

Any healthy diet needs commitment. And if you admit to a constant sweet tooth, you just need to dig deeper and constantly remind yourself of why you are embarking on this lifestyle journey. One of the first things you can do is keep a journal and study the times and situations that your sugar craving comes along. If you find that your sweet tooth acts up around three in the afternoon, you can fix yourself a healthy juice of fruits and vegetables before the clock hits three. Or you can schedule a workout around that time to get a natural dose of endorphins into your body.

There are also ten things you can do to satisfy your sweet cravings:

1. **Do not skip meals.** One of the worst things you can do is to send your blood sugar on a spiral by skipping meals. Eat right and eat on time.

2. **Use natural sweeteners.** The previous section gave many options on natural sweeteners that are rich in nutrients.
3. **Drink a lot of water.** We cannot stress it enough. Staying hydrated helps curb appetite and promotes good health.
4. **Drink fresh juice.** Freshly pressed fruits and vegetables (especially around the time you experience sweet cravings) curb appetite and give you a natural energy boost during the day.
5. **Plan your meals.** Invest the time to prepare your meals and fresh juicing ingredients the night before. Remember that no one can ever be too busy to prepare for a healthy lifestyle.
6. **Eat high fiber foods.** If you are already juicing, then you have got this one down! Fruits and vegetables are high in fiber, as well as in essential nutrients.
7. **Keep a clean pantry.** Healthy eating requires one hundred percent commitment. And it will not be fair if you do not spread the good habits you earn by eating well to your whole family. Rid your kitchen of junk food and processed foods, and fill your cupboards with healthy alternatives. Your kids might not be able to tell the difference.
8. **Get some exercise.** Studies have shown that exercising helps curb appetite. It also provides happy hormones in your body, much more fulfilling than eating a whole plate of cake.
9. **Walk away.** When everyone is eating all the "bad" foods, take a minute, drink a glass of water and walk away (for a minute or so). Binging might seem like a good idea, but you would be surprised how holding off will make you feel so much better afterwards.
10. **Stay committed.** Your primary motivation must be your own health. The secret to success of any lifestyle change is YOU.

This chapter has shown that there are ways to satisfy the urge for sugar without blowing your diet. We have come to understand why our bodies crave for sugar, and what we can do to control it. We have also learned about healthy alternatives that can replace sugar in our kitchen. Think about it: nature has given us so many sweeteners. Is it not about time that we take advantage of what has been given to us?

Chapter 12. Healthy Add-Ins

* * *

We have learned that drinking freshly pressed juices and blended smoothies is an easy and effective way of getting nutrition into your body. When taken fresh, these drinks turn into potent elixirs of vitamins, minerals, nutrients, enzymes, and antioxidants. Indeed, it is an effective way of protecting yourself against the toxins the modern world allows us to ingest.

Eating clean is not a fad. It is a way of life each and every person deserves because it is the way that we can enjoy our bodies. It is the road to living life to the fullest! While juices and smoothies have their share of critiques, it is undeniable that they are effective in helping the body absorb large amounts of nutrients. The enzymes then continue to aid digestion that, in turn, help our bodies digest food better and get more nutrients from what we consume.

But the health potential of juices and smoothies do not end there! Did you know that there are ingredients you can add to your juice or smoothie that add more super power to your drink? You can add them directly or you can use them as a topping. It works either way.

This chapter features a cheat sheet of ingredients you can add directly to your juice or smoothie. Get ready! You are about to meet a long list of super foods that will give your favorite beverage a bonus boost in health and nutrition!

Name of Add-In	What It Does For You
Coconut Oil	Coconut oil has a combination of fatty acids that have been proven for therapeutic effects. It is rich in medium chain triglycerides or MCTs that help protect against brain disorders. It is also good for the heart and strengthens your body against infections. Plus, it can make you eat less without trying because of ketone bodies that have an appetizing effect. You can even drink it before a workout to help you burn more fat.

	Add one to two tablespoons of coconut oil to your green smoothie to get the benefits of this super food into your system. You will not even notice the taste. But it might leave some clumps though. The trick is to melt the coconut oil a little and then add slowly to the smoothie. The possibilities do not end there. You can use coconut oil for hot drinks, baking, salads, frying, and cooking.
Chia Seeds	Chia seeds come from the chia plant. The nutrient content of this super food is simply mind-blowing. They are full of omega-three and omega-six fatty acids, dense with protein and fiber, and contain no cholesterol. Plus they have adequate amounts of calcium, potassium, copper, manganese, zinc, and phosphorus. You can imagine how much health benefits chia seeds can bring. They promote weight loss, increase energy, give pain relief, prevent heart disease, control blood sugar and blood pressure, reduce inflammation, aid digestion, and reduce bad cholesterol. Chia seeds have almost no flavor, so you can add them to any smoothie without changing the taste. But as a general guide, use one tablespoon for an eight-ounce glass by sprinkling them on or adding directly to the liquid. You can buy them in gel, powder, or whole-seed form.
Flax Seeds	A tablespoon of flaxseed will have about forty calories and three grams of fat. Now this is unsaturated fat we are talking about. It can help lower cholesterol levels and risk for heart disease. Talk about a nutrient boost! It also adds vitamins and minerals to your smoothie! Flaxseeds are rich in B complex vitamins, iron, and zinc that improve immunity. It is advisable to use ground flaxseed for your smoothie, rather than whole seeds. It is just easier to digest the powdered form. But if you buy them whole, simply run them through a coffee grinder before adding to your smoothie. Start with a small amount (about a teaspoon) and continue adding until you work your way up to a tablespoon.
Protein Powders	If you want a high-protein smoothie, consider adding whey

	protein into your smoothie. Fruit and vegetable drinks are great but they contain very little protein. Both meat-eaters and vegans will benefit from the protein content of whey protein. Protein is crucial in boosting the immune system and building muscle. It also gets absorbed into the blood stream faster— which makes it a great post-workout drink. One to two scoops into your smoothie will work well, plus it is relatively low in calories. Whey protein is definitely a good way to upgrade your healthy blend!
Hemp Seeds	Another great ingredient to add to your juice or smoothie is hemp seed. You usually buy this in powder form, and you add it directly to your beverage of choice. Hemp seeds are easily digestible and high in protein that does not cause bloating or gas (like some types of whey protein do). Not to mention in contains twenty amino acids and good fat! If you want to bulk up your immune system, you should strongly consider adding hemp seeds into your drink.
Mesquite	Mesquite is a nutritional powerhouse of protein, magnesium, calcium, zinc, iron, fiber, and lysine. More important, it is low on the glycemic index and good source of fiber. That means it digests slowly and does not cause a spike your blood sugar. One whiff of mesquite may get you hypnotized! It is sweet, nutty, smoky, and malty all at the same time. You can add it to your juice, smoothie, and raw desserts for that added oomph. Just one tablespoon is enough to add nutrition into your green smoothie. You can also sprinkle it on top of your hot beverage for added flavor.
Maca	Maca is a powerhouse of nutrition with admirable contents of vitamins B1, B2, B12, C, and E. It also has calcium, zinc, iron, magnesium, phosphorus, and amino acids. Plus it is high in protein and low in calories. It is an add-on that helps you keep calm, focused, and energized. Avid users also swear by its mood-lifting abilities.

	Here are a few more things you can expect maca to help you with: sex drive, fertility, memory, wound healing, improved immunity, stress relief; and support for your thyroid, pancreas, and thymus. The advice on using Maca is to start with small doses to your juice or smoothie. And do not consume more than two tablespoons daily.
Bee Pollen	Bee pollen is another miracle food you can sprinkle or add directly to your smoothie. Some people use them like candy, using them generously on cereals, yoghurts, and salads. What is bee pollen exactly? It is the male seed of a flower blossom gathered by the bees and mixed with the digestive enzymes of honeybees. It is the food of the young bee, and often called nature's most complete food. Bee pollen is rich in antioxidants, protein, and b-complex vitamins. It also has antibacterial, antifungal, and anti-inflammatory properties. Those with anemia, asthma, sinusitis, bronchitis, and constipation will benefit from adding bee pollen to their beverage. Studies show that athletes benefit from bee pollen as it improves performance and hastens recovery time.
Chlorella	Chlorella is often called a perfect food with good reason. In terms of nutrition content and health benefits, it is almost perfect. And it is widely used by both meat-eaters and vegetarians due to the non-animal source B vitamins found in chlorella. The green fresh-water algae contains vitamins B, C, E, K, beta-carotene, amino acids, magnesium, iron, carbohydrates, protein, and carbohydrates. And it has a wide range of health benefits—it improves digestion, reduces constipation, boosts immune system, relieves inflammation, reduces risk of cancer, cleanses the blood, reduces body odor, detoxifies against radiation, promotes tissue growth and repair.

	When starting with chlorella, add small quantities to your smoothie first. It initiates a detoxification process so nausea or diarrhea may be experienced. You may then increase the dose gradually.
Spirulina	If you have a sweet blend of fruit and veggie juice or smoothie, it might be a good opportunity to add spirulina to the mix. Spirulina does not taste good alone, so add fruits to mask its flavor.

Despite its pond water-like taste, it is amazingly good for you. It promotes dental health, boosts immunity, eliminates heavy metals from the body, and increases fat burn during exercise. Spirulina is a good source of protein, minerals, vitamins, and antioxidants. |
| Ginger | We have talked about the benefits of ginger early on, but it is worthwhile to discuss it again. Some people like adding it to their juice, while some have accustomed themselves to a ginger shot. A small dose of ginger can send warm feelings down your throat and awaken your senses!

Ginger contains potassium, sodium, iron, zinc, phosphorus, magnesium, copper, and calcium. It Is a well-known anti-inflammatory, anti-histamine, anti-septic, anti-viral, and a remedy to stomach pains and nausea.

Because it is anti-inflammatory, it is good for people who need to sooth muscle pain from rheumatism, arthritis, or strenuous physical activity. It also stimulates blood circulation and strengthens the overall immune system. |
| Cayenne | Adding cayenne pepper to your drink adds zing and nutrition to your drink. For many years, cayenne pepper has been known for its therapeutic properties that are effective against a wide range of disease.

Cayenne is dense in potassium, beta-carotene, calcium, B complex vitamins, and vitamins A, E, and C. It is good for the heart, in reducing risk of hypertension and cancer, lowering cholesterol, fighting infections, relieving arthritic pain, and aiding digestion problems. |

	It can also boost metabolism! Thinking of all that heat burning your fat away could be enough reason to down a few cayenne peppers today.
Savi Seeds	Savi seeds or sacha inchi seeds are star-shaped pods that resemble small nuts. You can eat them raw or bought in oil form. They taste wonderful so feel free to sprinkle them on your smoothie, salads, or eat raw as a snack. It has a nutty taste. Savi seeds are rich in antioxidants and essential fatty acids omega-three, omega-six, and omega-nine. Because of its high content of fatty acids, it promotes good mental health, it can lower blood sugar levels, protect against heart disease, and aids in weight loss.
Parsley	There was a time when parsley provided décor for plates of food. But it is no longer just a table garnish. Parsley contains two components that do the body good. The first is a volatile oil that includes myristicin, limonene, eugenol, and alpha-thujene. And the second is flavonoids, including apiin, apigenin, crisoeriol, and luteolin. These are a rich source of antioxidants! Parsley has a vibrant flavor and healing properties. It contains folate, iron, and vitamins B, K, C, and A. Add this to your drink if you want to flush out excess water from your body, control your blood pressure, relax muscles, boost immunity, and reduce your risk of cancer.
Cilantro	Cilantro is known to be effective as a natural cleansing agent. It helps the body cleanse itself of toxic metals that bind to tissue. Those who have reported mercury exposures have benefited from ingesting regular amounts of cilantro. Cilantro is rich in vital vitamins A, K, and C, folic acid, riboflavin, niacin, and beta-carotene. It is high in phytonutrients that fight off a long list of chronic diseases. Cilantro reduces anxiety, fights disease, improves sleep, can lower sugar, and prevents cardiovascular damage. Those with

	Alzheimer's, Parkinson's, arthritis, diabetes, autism, Tourette syndrome, Bell's Palsy, and infertility benefit from the herb as well.

Speaking of heart, you have to be warned that cilantro is not for the faint of heart. It adds a very distinct flavor that might take some getting used to. |
| Basil | While many love basil with their sandwiches, burgers, pizza, salads, and dishes, health-enthusiasts are going crazy over basil too.

Basil contains high levels of vitamin A, lutein, zea-xanthin, cryptoxanthin, and beta-carotene. It is a known anti-oxidant, anti-microbial, and anti-viral.

Its health benefits make it even more worthwhile to add into juices. Studies show that it has the potential to fight cancer. It also helps you think clearly by promoting blood circulation in the brain. And many have been using it to those with attention deficit disorders and ADHD.

If you would like to try juicing basil, one-fourth of your brew should consist of the herb. Enjoy experimenting the flavor with different fruits and vegetables. |
| Turmeric | Turmeric is soothing as a hot beverage! You can also add it to your fruit and vegetable juice and smoothies. Many people are enjoying fresh turmeric juice because of its many healing properties.

Turmeric is anti-microbial, attacking bacterial and viral infections. And if you are always dealing with respiratory tract infections and autoimmune disease, turmeric will help you get over that cold or fly in no time.

It is also a potent cancer fighter, a natural liver detoxifier, slows the progression of Alzheimer's disease, and fights allergies and congestion.

And the best part of all, turmeric speeds up metabolism and |

	burns fat. But like all ingredients, it is always best to start slow and work your way up in terms of the amount of turmeric you put. Start with a teaspoon and see how your body reacts to it.
Lucuma Root	If you confess to having a sweet tooth, and if you like chocolate, vanilla, or caramel—you would warm up to the flavor of the lucuma root in no time. Lucuma comes from a Peruvian fruit, known as "The Gold of the Incas". In fact, it is the most popular ice cream flavor in Peru! Lucuma is perfect for smoothies, cookies, brownies, cheesecake, and ice cream. You get the picture of how good it is, right? Apart from being a natural sweetener, it is loaded with nutrients, vitamin B, zinc, calcium, iron, fiber, complex carbohydrates, and antioxidants such as beta-carotene. Needless to say, it abounds with health benefits. It boosts vitality, relieves symptoms of fatigue, promotes bone health, helps resolve digestive issues, and has a low GI content.

It is absolutely amazing how nature has provided us all these super foods! We literally have good health and nutrition at our fingertips. It is unfortunate that society has not trained us to reach for these. And instead, we live in a world consumed by sugar, fat, preservatives, and toxins. But the good news is that there is always an opportunity to start over and make a choice towards a healthy lifestyle!

Fresh fruits and vegetable juices and smoothies are already very healthy. Who would have thought that adding one to two tablespoons of simple and natural ingredients could boost the nutrient content of your health tonic further? Your next move would be to head out at your nearest whole foods store and get your self to the super foods aisle.

Conclusion

* * *

We live in a world consumed by a diet of fat, processed foods, preservatives, and countless toxic substances. Scientific research is showing that majority of people have an internal cocktail of toxic chemicals that confuse our body, result in imbalance, and lead to an array of chronic diseases. Come to think of it, there has never been a time when the incidences of obesity, cancer, and cardiovascular disease have become so rampant.

If there is one thing we have learned, it is that cure and prevention is within reach. We simply have to look at fruits, vegetables, herbs, nuts, and seeds to provide us with potent nutrients and anti-oxidants that can build the foundation of a strong and healthy life. Every trip to the market and the grocery can become your health revolution. And all you need is your juicer to get started!

If you have picked up this e-book, it means you are ready to take back your health and heal yourself through natural alternatives. And with the knowledge the past thirteen chapters have shared with you, I am sure you are now well on your way to being a pro in juicing fresh fruits and vegetables!

Apples, Carrots and Kale-Oh My! Now we know that there are so much more of nature's best and freshest goods that we can add to juice blends. And these are sure to be so good that you will not help but say "Oh My!".

Juices pressed from fruits and vegetables are not only delicious, they are super healthy. In its juice form, vitamins and minerals are easily digested and absorbed, allowing our bodies to maximize the nutrients and antioxidants nature meant for us to receive. In fact this e-book has brought us through lists after lists of ingredients that has jotted down all the antioxidants and phytonutrients there are! And much more, they are effective fighters of the common diseases we have today due to an unhealthy lifestyle.

So what are you waiting for? Ready, press, juice!

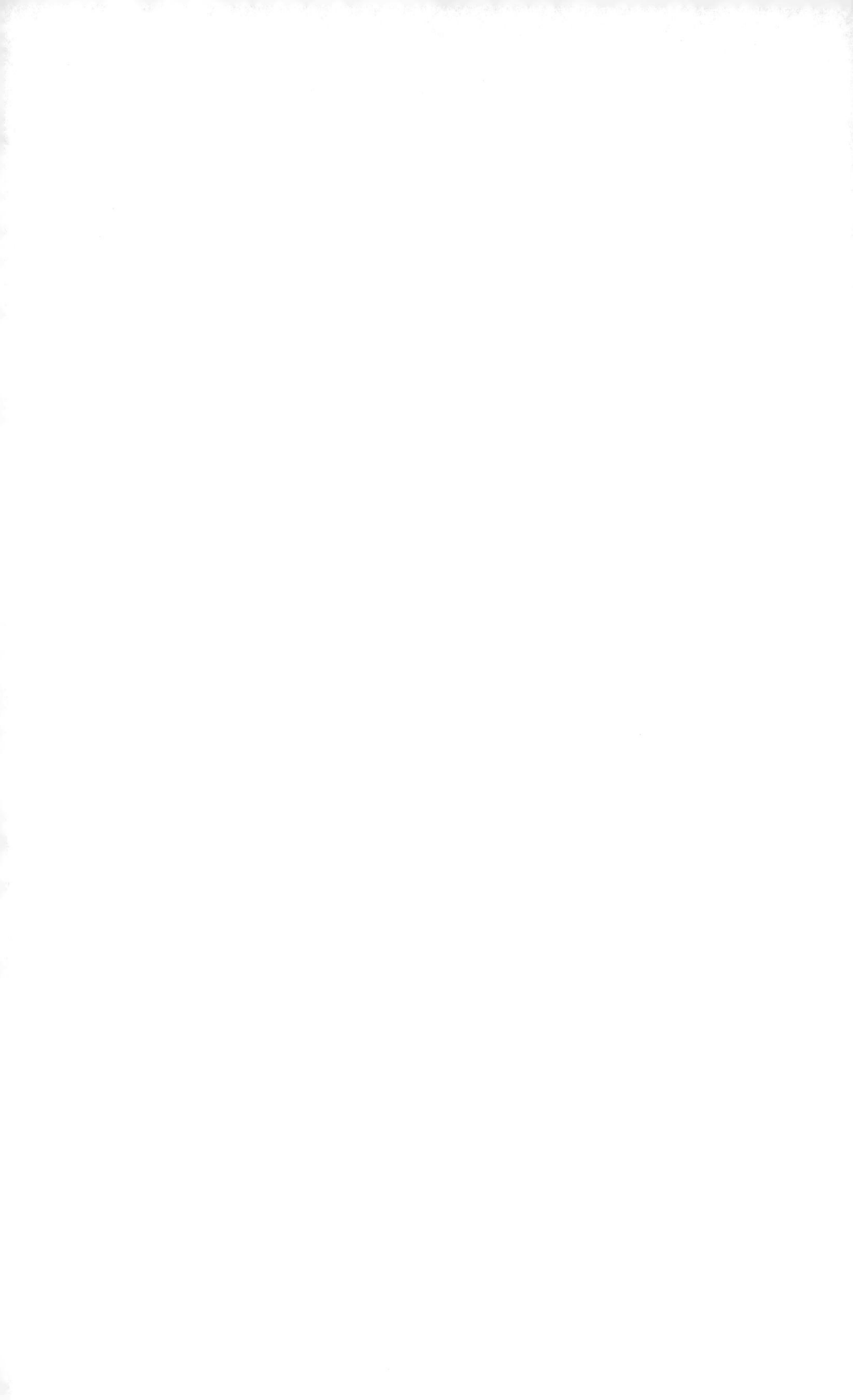